FORGOTTEN GIRL

*A powerful true story of amnesia,
secrets and second chances*

NAOMI JACOBS

PAN BOOKS

First published 2015 by Pan Books
an imprint of Pan Macmillan, a division of Macmillan Publishers Limited
Pan Macmillan, 20 New Wharf Road, London N1 9RR
Basingstoke and Oxford
Associated companies throughout the world
www.panmacmillan.com

ISBN 978-1-4472-8272-3

1 3 5 7 9 8 6 4 2

A CIP catalogue record for this book is available from the British Library.

Printed and bound by CPI Group (UK) Ltd, Croydon, CR0 4YY

FORGOTTEN GIRL

For Simone, Katie and Leo –
this wouldn't have happened without your love

CONTENTS

1
Not in Kansas Anymore

You follow the rainbow
in the hope of someday finding
that pot of gold at the end.
One day maybe.
One day.

R. D.

I stood still, staring at the classroom door.

There was a bag on my shoulder and a small pot, mud-brown and lidded, in my hand.

Pride surged through me. I had made this pot all by myself. I knocked on the door and an unfamiliar voice told me to enter.

A wooden stool stood in the corner and I walked to it and sat down. The woman sitting opposite was a teacher; I knew her name was Rebecca and she wasn't from my school, but she was there to see me.

Her face was framed by masses of curly brown hair. She pursed her lips, took the pot from my hand, and placed it on the table next to her. It was home to pots of all different shapes and sizes, a sea of vibrant colour. The larger ones were adorned with small pieces of broken mirror, azure seascapes and purple-orange skies. The smaller ones had silver-glittered necks, gold hieroglyphs, and small red lids. It was a dazzling display of pottery perfection. In the middle sat my pot: forlorn, pathetic, brown, and very plain.

'You've failed.' She shot me a disappointed look.

'What? No way!' I said.

I glanced at my pot and it looked back at me apologetically. 'But I worked really hard on it.'

'That may be, but I can't pass you. You've failed. Look, it's not nearly as good as the others.'

I knew she was right. They were the older, more attractive siblings, possessing a creative beauty that my runt-of-the-litter pot could not live up to. I thought about the hard work I had put into it and, as if on cue, a volcanic fear of failure erupted within me. The force of this made me jump from my stool, grab my bag, and run out of the door.

In another classroom, along a deserted corridor, my friends were sitting at their desks talking to each other. I tried the door handle but it was locked. I banged on the glass, calling to them to let me in. Nobody turned round. Instead, I watched as they laughed among themselves.

'Guys, it's me: Nay. Open the door!'

One by one, they raised their heads and stared at me. My best friend Katie appeared at the glass pane. 'Open the door,' I demanded, rattling the handle. 'I need to get in.' Laughing, Katie shook her head and pointed up at a clock on the classroom wall where black hands were ticking slowly over Roman numerals. She walked across to the blackboard and chalked up the word *échec*. It was French for 'failure'. Everyone was watching her and laughing. I banged my fist against the glass again in despair. Suddenly I heard shouts coming from the far end of the corridor. The Mega Smegs – girls from our year whom we loathed – were running at me, chanting, 'Failure, failure, failure . . .'

I turned back to the door. My friends were gone and the room was filling with clocks – hundreds of them, all over the desks, the walls; different sizes, different kinds. Grand-dad clocks, cuckoo clocks, alarm clocks. Then, just as they appeared, they all started to fade.

'You have to get Leo,' a voice whispered.

As the girls came closer I felt my body vibrating and shaking with fear. I turned and ran towards a pair of double doors at the other end of the corridor.

I had no choice. I pushed them open.

I stepped into a bright, burning light.

Clutching my chest, furiously grabbing for air, I sat up in bed. I couldn't breathe. Gulping down sobs, I tried to scream. Nothing came.

There was a small window opposite the bed. I looked up at it, willing my breathing to calm. The sun shone cheerfully through the curtains, illuminating the purple flowers covering them. *Purple flowers?*

I closed my eyes. 'S'okay, Nay, it's just a dream,' I said out loud.

I grabbed my throat. My voice sounded . . . weird, different; hoarse and deep. Like a grown-up's. I opened my eyes and scanned the room, turning my head slowly to the left and then to the right. Nothing. I recognized nothing. I looked down at my body. The pyjama top I was wearing was drenched with sweat. I tried to think and my head started to hurt. This wasn't my bunk bed. Where was my Marilyn Monroe duvet cover? This wasn't the bedroom I shared with my sister. Where was she? Where was Simone? I closed my eyes again.

'I must be dreaming,' I said to the empty room. My voice again; it sounded so strange. I jumped out of the weirdly large bed. Had it kidnapped me in my sleep and brought me to this strange place? I looked around at the room. It was dismal and grey. There was no carpet on the floor, just bare boards, and the walls had been stripped down to bare grey plaster. It looked almost like a prison.

I walked slowly out of the room into the hallway, hoping I would see something familiar. The house felt empty. 'Hello,' I called out. To the left of me was a closed bedroom door but in front of me was a bathroom; the door was ajar. I pushed it open. No one was in there and I didn't recognize anything inside. There was a mirror above the sink. *Maybe*, I thought, *if I see my reflection I will know that I am still dreaming and wake up.*

It took a slow second, but when my mouth dropped open in horror, I grabbed my face and screamed, 'NO! Oh my God, oh my God oh my God oh my God . . . I'm . . . I'm . . . I'm OLD!!' I was *old*.

Shock made me back away from the mirror. I burst into tears and dropped to the floor. My brain tried to make sense of the face I had just seen, asking what was with the lines? The dark circles under my eyes and the short hair? No, no, it wasn't me. I jumped up from the floor and stared at the face again. 'This isn't me!' I shouted at it.

I ran back into the bedroom, shaken by what I had seen. I felt a cold panic box its way into my mind, punching tiny holes of anxiety into my brain. Dread found its place. Where was my sister? I felt the sudden urge to find her. Maybe she was in the living room.

Panicked, I sped downstairs and stormed into an unfamiliar kitchen. Nothing. I ran back into the living room. No one.

I flew back upstairs and, avoiding the other closed door down the small hallway, I rushed into the bedroom and flung open the wardrobe doors, looking for one of my smeghead* friends maybe, who would yell, 'Surprise!' and keel over laughing at the crap joke she was playing.

'Oh. My. Dayz,' I gasped.

The colours were unbelievable: blues, purples, yellows, but . . . like . . . different. Clothes I would never wear. 'This isn't my house.' I shook my head at them. I spun around. 'This isn't my room . . . This is NOT my life. NO!' I ran back into the bathroom and looked at the face again. 'This isn't me!' I shouted back at it. Dizzy, I hit the floor. My body curled up into a ball and I started to cry again. I tried to find something to focus my mind on, anything, and then I remembered that I had seen a picture of my sister downstairs. But I didn't get up; I just lay there, crying, moaning, and mumbling.

After lying there for what felt like ages, I realized that I

---

* *Smeghead* – complete and total (usually quite ignorant) idiot, who has no clue about anything outside of his/her own head. A popular swear word from the BBC2 TV series *Red Dwarf*.

wasn't dreaming. This was real; I was real. I had woken up in a bed I didn't know, a room I didn't recognize, and a house that wasn't mine.

And then I heard music in the distance, a song being sung. I crawled across the bathroom floor and back into the bedroom while a woman sang something about bleeding or breathing; no, it was definitely bleeding, yes, bleeding love. The music was coming from something on the bedside cabinet. It kept stopping and starting and stopping again; but there was no radio, no tape deck, just a small black object shaking violently across the top.

I jumped back, almost falling over myself. The sound hurt my ears and as I cautiously picked it up, the word 'Simone' flashed in black letters.

'Simone?' I asked it.

Simone! It was my sister; it had to be. She was the only Simone I knew. I turned the strange object over and over, pressing hard plastic. There were no buttons. I put it up to my mouth and called Simone's name, hoping she would somehow hear me. The flashing, the music and the vibrating stopped. 'Where are the frickin' buttons?' I screamed at it, and a great sense of inadequacy produced even more tears. I felt defeated. 'Three missed calls' it now read.

'What the . . . ? This, like . . . is this a phone?'

I dropped the phone on the floor, ran down the stairs to the front door, and stepped outside. The houses opposite stared at me; their windows looked like laughing eyes. Frantically, I scanned the tree-lined road. I didn't know what I was looking for, but I so knew this wasn't Wolverhampton. This wasn't my home town. I didn't live here. A woman walking a small white dog passed the hedge separating the front garden from the road and smiled at me. I turned away. I must have looked such a div standing in the garden in my pyjamas.

I ran back into the house, slammed the door shut and stood facing the stairs. My heart was thundering in my chest. I closed my eyes and counted to ten and as my breathing slowed down, I grabbed my forehead with both hands. 'Come on, Nay.' I took another deep breath. 'You're all right, girl. Everything's gonna be okay; you just need to chill the smeg out.'

Through deep breaths and several counts of ten, I talked myself into some semblance of calm. For the first time, I saw the different-sized photos hanging on the walls on either side of the stairs. I started with the ones closest to me, pictures of this chubby baby with a cute smile and a head of brown kiss curls. My brain was saying, 'Leo,' but I didn't know who he was. The next set of frames answered my question – they showed me but older, me smiling back with a chubby toddler on my lap.

Was this really *me*? Was this child *mine*? Is this *the future*?

Trying to think instantly caused a bright light to flash in front of my eyes and a stabbing pain to shoot through my head. I took another deep breath. The pain subsided and I climbed two more steps. The next picture was of Simone proudly holding a white scroll, a black gown draped over her shoulders, a black cap on her head. 'You went to uni? When did this happen?' I asked the photo. Maybe I was in my sister's house, I thought.

I looked at the rest of the pictures, more pictures of this child I instinctively knew was called Leo. He grew with each photograph and the last one was a black-and-white one of him holding a skateboard. The smile, the eyes . . . it was like looking at a mini version of me. *Maybe he's my brother?* I wondered if my mum had had another kid.

I searched the other pictures to see if there was any hint of his mum; no, if he wasn't with me, he was on his own. Photographs of my sister sat next to pictures of my father. I stood staring at his face in shock. Was it really him? In one of the photographs he was with another child I didn't recognize. He was lighter in skin tone, with straw-blond hair, and he looked a bit like Simone.

'What year is this?' I asked the pictures. Nothing, no answer. I stepped backwards down the stairs and made my way into the living room, desperately trying to remember something. A black cordless phone sat near the television and as soon as I looked at it, a number popped into my head.

I continued to pace, stopped, looked back at the phone and heard the number again.

7768339, this time with a name: *Katie*.

'Katie?' I asked the phone. The number came to me again. *7768339, Katie.*

It was a strange-looking phone with no pull-out aerial and it had an orange screen, but every time I looked at it, I kept getting the same name and number. *7768339, Katie.* Katie from school?

The only way to find out was to press the numbers. It rang about four times and then someone answered.

'Hello,' a soft, high-pitched voice sang into the phone.

'Hello,' I whispered. 'Is that you, Kate?'

'Oh, hiya, babe. I was just about to call you. Did you manage to sleep last night?'

She knew me. 'Katie?' I asked again. This wasn't my friend from school. This Katie sounded as old as my mum and like she had just stepped off *Coronation Street*.

'Yeah.' She went quiet for a moment. 'What's up, hun? Are you okay?'

The gates opened, allowing a flash flood of tears. 'Oh my God,' I sobbed. 'I don't know who you are. I don't know where I am and this number kept repeating over and over in my head so I called you, and it's not you. And I don't know what to do and I don't know where I . . . and I don't know who you are, and I don't know what's happened to my face.'

'Your face? What's happened to your face?' The strange woman's voice went up an octave.

'IT'S OLD!' I began to cry again.

'What?' She laughed and then went silent again. 'Naomi, what's wrong? Erm, okay, okay, babe, listen to me, take a deep breath.'

I sobbed some more; this definitely wasn't Katie from school.

'But I don't know you,' I managed.

'Right, okay, listen to me,' she said in a deliberately calm voice. 'Go into the kitchen, switch the kettle on and make yourself a cup of coffee.'

'C . . . coffee?' I stammered. 'Ugh, gross.'

She went quiet again.

'Hello?' I walked into the kitchen anyway, searched for the kettle, and switched it on.

'Erm, I'm here, babe. Listen, Gerald's getting the car out the garage, and we'll be round in five minutes. Have you found the kettle?'

'Hmm.' I opened up the cupboard in front of me. A range of coffees and boxes of herbal teas stood on display.

'Right, make yourself a cuppa. You like herbal teas, don't you?'

'Yes,' I replied.

'Okay, right. Make yourself a tea, and have a cigarette, and we'll be round in a bit.'

'Cigarette? Rank! I *sooooo* don't smoke.'

The silence was so long, I thought she had hung up. Had I said something wrong? I started to cry again. 'I don't know jack about anything. I don't know what I'm doing here.'

'It's okay. Right, right, just . . . just breathe and . . . and drink your tea. I'm coming round, okay?'

'Okay.'

I put the phone down. The fresh minty smell of the tea kinda reminded me of my stepfather, Joseph. It was his favourite tea and he used to slurp it loudly knowing it would make me laugh. I began to wonder why there were no pictures of him on the wall, or of my mum. Where *was* everybody?

The warmth of the tea comforted me. As I held the cup between my hands, I decided I liked the kitchen. The bright orange and yellow walls held pictures painted by a child – probably, I thought, the one from the photographs. Certificates and postcards surrounded the artwork. On the white door of one of the cupboards was an Irish blessing, a picture of a lone castle with nothing but blue skies, green hills and brown boulders of rock around it. Above the castle were the words:

When times are hard
May your heart never
Turn to stone.
When shadows
Fall on you
Remember,
You never walk
alone.

Everything seemed to, like, for a minute . . . chill. I needed to let go of the sheer terror of what I was experiencing. The blessing gave me a moment of freedom from the deep shudders of panic that kept sending massive waves of distress through my body, forcing it to flood with adrenaline, making me want to run. I was exhausted. So I let go of the urgent need to know where, when and who I was. In that moment, I was sure I would eventually find my way home, back to 1992 and out of this nightmare.

The doorbell rang. I took a deep breath. Once I opened that door, I would be faced with yet more of the unknown. I hadn't a clue what was happening. But I knew two things for sure:

1. I was fifteen years old.
2. I had woken up in the future.

2
The Future

A
journey of
a thousand miles starts
beneath one's feet

L. T. E.

I mentally took the brace position as I opened the front door. A short, strawberry-blonde-haired woman, her face full of concern, stepped towards me.

'You all right?'

I stared raw-eyed and shook my head, thinking that this was totally mental. This was definitely not my school friend Katie. In fact, this colourfully dressed woman with her silver jewellery and suede tasselled bag was the complete opposite. I backed away from her.

'Naomi, love, can I come in?' she asked gently.

I want to go home, I thought, as she followed me into the living room and took my hand.

'Are you all right, babe?'

The tears flowed thick and fast. I could only shake my head again.

'What's happened?'

I opened my mouth but it had suddenly stopped working. I was frickin' speechless.

'You know who I am, right?'

I gave her a blank look and rubbed my forehead. My head was still hurting, thumping with pain.

'Naomi, I'm your friend, Katie. We've known each other for five years. Look.' She turned to the window and pointed to the red car sitting outside the house. 'That lump o' lard is his highness, Gerald.' She turned back to me, smiling. 'Loves his food, his ale, and me. I've got four kids, remember? Alex, Dylan, Adam and Chloe and we . . .' She stopped and took a look around. 'Is Leo at school?'

'Leo?'

'Yes, hun, Leo.' She gave me a strange look. 'Your son.'

I had guessed right then. Leo was the chubby-faced, yogurt-covered kid in the photograph on the kitchen wall.

'He must be at school right now.' She looked around the room as if I might have stashed him somewhere.

This was information I couldn't process, yet couldn't deny. Stuck in a sort of maternal limbo, I did have a sense that my body had had a child, but trying to remember him made my head hurt again. I rubbed my temples and thought instead, *That'll be why these boobs look like they could hold a smeggin' pencil case, never mind a pencil*. But wait, she'd asked me some questions, hadn't she?

'I think I remember you. I don't know where Leo is.' I looked at her. 'I don't remember.'

I pulled my hand from hers, trying to forget the let's-test-the-pertness-of-your-boobs-with-a-pencil test the girls and I had done in the P.E. changing rooms.

'Tell you what, why don't you come to mine for a cuppa and we'll figure this all out. Let's get you dressed.'

I stopped pacing and stared at her. I was scared, I was confused, I wanted her help, but she was a stranger.

'Come on.' I followed her up to the bedroom and watched her from the doorway as she opened the purple-flowered curtains, allowing a dim light in.

'Clothes!' she exclaimed cheerfully as if they were the answer to all my problems. We both looked at the white wardrobe stood in the corner. She pulled open the doors and went through the rack of garms* bulging from their wooden home.

This Katie was dressed a bit like a hippie, with a long black skirt, green kaftan top, beaded and crystal jewellery and loads of silver rings of all different shapes and sizes. With her full breasts, small hips and long unkempt hair, she kinda looked like an earth-mothery type. I relaxed a bit when I realized that this woman was not here to harm me.

She pulled out a wine-coloured velour tracksuit and held it up. 'This one.'

I tried to stop myself from laughing and ended up snorting like Miss Piggy. The clothes were majorly offensive.

'What?' She looked from me to the criminal piece of clothing and smiled. 'What's wrong with it?'

'Are you smeggin' mental? Whose trackie is *that*?'

'It's the fashion,' she sighed.

---

* *Garms* – many items of clothing (garments).

'Yeah, like in the seventies maybe,' I snorted. 'That is *sooooo* making me wanna barf.'

'Barf?' She was clueless.

'Hurl, spew, chuck . . . throw up?'

'Oh.' She burst out laughing. 'I don't get the tracksuit thing myself; it's all a bit Crockett and Tubbs for me.'

I gave her a small smile. Even though she was old, she seemed okay. I stepped fully into the bedroom and edged closer to her.

Katie put the tracksuit back in the wardrobe. 'Not doing a *Miami Vice* then,' she told it, and pulled out a large black jumper instead. 'There you go, plain and simple.'

She closed the mirrored doors and I saw that old face again, my face, and felt panic twist in the pit of my stomach. She noticed my horrified reaction and put her hand on my shoulder. 'Naomi, everything's gonna be all right, you know?'

'I know,' I said, nodding. 'I can borrow Eve's Oil of Ulay.'

Her smile dropped slightly when I said my mum's name, but I blanked it, pulling the jumper off the hanger to put it up against my wiry frame. 'Have I got jeans or a skirt or sumthin'?'

'I think you wear it with tights.' She opened the top drawer of the chest of drawers standing behind her.

'It's a dress?' My jaw dropped.

She smiled. 'There you go.' She handed me a pair of tights.

I stared at them, stunned by the aqua green-blue nylon shimmer; the colour was almost unreal, acieed* trippy unreal. I had never seen anything like it before.

---

* *Acieed* – a word taken from 'We Call It Acieed' by D-Mob (a popular 80s tune).

'Come on.' She woke me from my fashion daze. 'I'll wait downstairs for you.'

I got washed and dressed quick time, avoiding the mirrors. Instead, I concentrated on the clothes, thinking, *We used to wear jumper dresses when I was, like, ten! Is this the eighties? What's going on?*

Downstairs, Katie was holding a pair of black sheepskin-lined boots. I raised my eyebrows and turned my mouth in disgust.

'They're your Ugg boots,' she said.

'Ugh.' They were even worse than the tracksuit. 'Is that, like, short for "Ugly"? Is this a joke?' I looked around for the hidden camera, as this was beyond the realm of mental.

She burst out laughing. 'Everyone wears them; try them on.'

I hesitated. Then reckoned if she was my spar* like she said she was, then surely she wouldn't let me leave the house looking like a total div? I grabbed them from her, put them on, and found they were warm and comfy.

'Come on. Ged's waiting.' When she opened the front door my stomach started to flip and I sucked in my breath. I was frozen again, unable to move.

'No, I can't. I don't want to.' I stared out into the street. It was quiet except for the rumbling traffic in the distance.

She grasped hold of my hand. 'Naomi, look at me. I will not let anything happen to you. You will be safe with me.' She said each word slowly, making sure I heard every last syllable.

---

* *Spar* – a really good friend who wouldn't allow you to commit a fashion faux pas.

'I know you don't remember anything right now,' she contin-ued, 'but one day, I promise, one day you will and, until that day, I will make sure you are okay. Okay?'

The look of sincerity in her eyes seemed to coax my fears out from a small corner of mistrust and into a space of accept-ance. I nodded and hung my head, relief flooding over me. She put her arms around me and I let her hug me, feeling safe. As long as I had this friendly, calm, patient woman around, things wouldn't feel so . . . stale*.

This woman, who was called Katie but was not my friend from school, gently wiped my face and then beckoned me to the car. She grabbed some keys from the hook on the wall and closed the front door. Her husband gave me a friendly smile, jumped out of the driver's seat, and opened the back door for me.

As the car pulled away, I stared out of the window at the unfamiliar house in which I had woken up. It was a small, brown-brick two-up two-down, with a tiny garden at the front. It was my own house of horrors, the last ride of the trav-elling funfair that stopped entertaining the moment I found myself trapped in it. Katie turned in her seat. 'I've called your sister, hun. She's on her way.'

We pulled up into the drive of a terraced, newly built, three-storey grey and white house. I got out of the car and stared down the long cul-de-sac, not recognizing anything.

'We've been here about three months. Four bedrooms, three floors,' Katie informed me as I followed her through the

---

* *Stale* – really bad (nothing to do with bread).

hallway into the kitchen. 'And this is my domain,' she said proudly.

The kitchen was light and airy and very large, with a big dining table and a brown leather sofa at one side. I could smell a faint aroma of sweet incense; in the corners were exotic-looking plants and glacial crystals. The walls were covered with crayon drawings of angels, dolphins, rainbows and robots. It was warm and inviting.

'Sit down, babe. I'll stick the kettle on.'

I sank into the sofa; it was comfortable. On the other side of the large patio doors a gigantic, fat cherry-wood Buddha sat facing me. I felt like it was laughing at me.

'When's my sister getting here?'

'She'll be here soon. She's not far. She's left work early but it's on the other side of town so . . . She'll be here soon, babe. Naomi, do you know where we are?'

I nodded. 'Yeah, Manchester.' *Wow! What? Wait!* I thought. How did I know this all of a sudden? Katie asked me more questions. How long had I been living in the city? Yes! I knew the name of the road and the number of the house I had woken up in. I was flummoxed. How did I know this? I didn't know it when I woke up. I tried to remember moving into the house or the first time I arrived in Manchester.

Nothing.

'But when I woke up, I didn't know where I was, or how I got here, and it's like I know where I am now, but I can't remember living here.' I was so confused.

'So what's the last thing you do remember?' she asked.

I looked into the drink she had handed me, hoping to see a reflection or an image of my life. I saw my pink and white bedroom in our house in Wolverhampton. I saw the small red-brick terraced house I shared with my younger sister, my mum, and my stepfather. I closed my eyes and clasped the cup in my hands. All I could see was me in my bed, late at night. I could hear my mum watching TV downstairs. Simone was on the top bunk bed above me, snoring quietly, while I was under the blankets with my trusty torch reading a French GCSE revision book and thinking about Robert Harris, the totally fit boy I fancied, but who didn't fancy me back.

'I fell asleep and . . .' I paused. 'I woke up in the future.'

'Do you know how old you are?' Katie was staring at me, wide-eyed, like an owl.

'Fifteen, I think, but I know I'm not. I know I'm old.'

Katie laughed. 'God, if you're old, then I'm ancient; you're only thirty-two.'

I smiled, but it so wasn't funny. Thirty *was* ancient. After that, you were cashing in your pension.

I took a sip of the coffee. It tasted awful, bitter and acidic. 'Gross, Mr Morose,' I muttered. 'Do I like coffee?' I asked her. 'I mean, who would, like, really drink this?'

'Well.' She hesitated. 'You do, in fact. You drink it all the time.'

I didn't understand and Katie looked confused. But hey, I just didn't like coffee. I decided not to go there. Instead, I tried to remember something, but the pain just kept kicking my brain around my skull like John Barnes with a football.

When she asked certain questions, I found I was able to answer them easily. I knew my date of birth, my age, my address, my postcode, Leo's name, Katie's telephone number, specific details about this life. I even knew it was Thursday

17 April and it was 2008. But what I did for my last birthday? No. How I met Katie? Nothing. What happened at the birth of Leo? Nada. I couldn't find the memories anywhere in my mind.

'When I look too hard, I get, like, this white-hot burning sensation that slaps my temples silly and shakes my head into, like, a dizzy spazoid meltdown. It seriously just makes me wanna hit the deck, and hurl again.'

'I have no clue what you just said then.' Katie gave a nervous laugh and shook her head. 'I think . . . just . . . don't try and remember now; I'm sure it will come to you.'

She didn't look so sure. Neither was I, and in that moment I decided that I would use all of my brainpower to will myself to fall asleep that night and wake up the next day back in my bunk bed, safe, secure, still fifteen and still thinking only of school, exams, and totally fit Robert Harris. Yes, back to 1992.

As we were talking, the doorbell rang and Katie got up to answer it. It was my sister, I knew it was, but at this moment, I was afraid to see her. The last thing I remembered of my fourteen-year-old sister was that we had been arguing over hair gel and insulting each other in the worst ways imaginable. Should I believe the photos on the walls in that house? How much had she changed? Did she look old? Were we close or distant? Would she believe me? Could she help me? Would she tell Mum and Dad? Cause I *sooooo* didn't want her to.

As she walked into the kitchen, I freaked out. She wasn't the Simone I knew but I could tell it was her. She was taller but still shorter than me, the corkscrew curls in her hair were now straight and she had gone kind of chubby.

Wait. How had this happened? I thought. How had I

gone skinny and she gone podgy? Simone still had the same almond-shaped soft brown eyes with fine eyelashes, straight nose, and full lips. Her smile was still large and beautiful and . . . she wasn't wearing braces.

What? She's had her braces off? NO WAY! I touched my teeth and realized that I had also.

And then it hit me like a ton of bricks.

This really is the future.

When I realized the gap in memory was so huge and I had missed seventeen years of loving my sister, I burst into tears. She came straight to me and gave me one of her infamous hugs. Her backbreaking, oxygen-squeezing, I-really-love-you hugs, and as she held me tight, I knew beyond a shadow of a doubt that it was Simone. My beautiful, loving, kind but tough as* sister. I sobbed into her embrace.

'It's okay, *chica*,' she said gently, taking a step back and wiping my soaked face. 'What's happened, babe?' Tears welled in her eyes.

'I don't know, Sim, I don't know.' I couldn't breathe. 'My brain's gone anal and it's, like, crapping itself!' I grabbed my head. 'And I've got blue tights.' I pointed at my knees. 'Oh my God. Look at you!' I laughed and pointed at her. 'I feel sick.'

I wiped away my tears, took a deep breath, and went over everything since I had woken up in the future, trying to leave nothing out. My sister listened intently. She became more

---

* *Tough as* – as tough as nails, old boots, or any other hard object (another way of saying you wouldn't mess with someone in a fight because they are really hard!)

serious as I told her about waking up in that house and not remembering how I got there, but she didn't say a word.

When I finished, she looked at Katie then turned to me. 'You remember me, right?'

'No, not really. Not like you are now.'

'It's okay, babe. It will be okay. I think we should call your doctor. Do you know the number?'

I shook my head.

'What about your mobile?' she asked.

'My what? Why the smeg would I have a baby toy?'

Simone looked at Katie. 'Your mobile phone? It should have all of your numbers in it.'

I had no idea what they were talking about. Maybe it was that strange-looking cordless phone at the house.

'It's at the house . . . I think.'

'I'll send Ged for it,' Katie said.

Like a sergeant major pulling troops together, Simone's voice changed to the familiar tone of someone taking charge. 'Okay, and we'll call the doctor and get you in, see if he can figure out what's happening.'

'What about taking her to the hospital?' Katie suggested.

'NO!' I bellowed. 'Don't take me to the hospital. I won't go, and you can't frickin' make me!' Images of doctors telling me it was a brain tumour or some deadly brain disease suddenly had me wanting to fight anyone who might force me to step inside an A&E. Besides, later, under the cover of darkness, I was going back to 1992 so it didn't matter.

'I'll go to the doctor's. It's not that serious.'

While Ged went to fetch my 'mobile phone', Simone and Katie started discussing what could possibly be wrong with me. The conversation between them was interjected with questions to me about whether I had possibly wrapped up* and banged my head without knowing it. Trying to remember anything was still causing me major pain so they stopped asking me questions. Instead, sensing I couldn't take too much in, they gave me the basics, explaining about Leo while I just listened, a little fascinated about a life I had no clue about. This helped to stop the searing pain and I began to separate my mind from the person they were telling me about. They were talking about someone else, someone I didn't know. They were talking about Adult Naomi.

I didn't ask that many questions. I was too afraid to know why certain faces were missing from the wall of photographs, namely my mother and my stepfather. I waited for Simone to mention them and she didn't, so I decided I didn't need to know, because maybe they had left us like I always thought they would. Anyway, it was Adult Naomi's business, not mine, but . . .

Having a child at twenty-one years of age? What was that about? I couldn't believe it. I wondered whether she was totally off her head. That's too young to be having a kid. I mean, I had babysat for kids since I was twelve, but no way was I gonna have any.

Unless I was getting paid to babysit, I *sooooo* didn't do children! To be told Adult Naomi did, and quite early on in her life, was totally incomprehensible. I was also majorly disappointed to learn that the house I had woken up in was in fact her two-bedroom council house that she shared with her

---

* *Wrap up* – fall over/fall down (nothing to do with scarves or winter).

son. I did *not* want to know how she'd ended up living there. In fact, there wasn't much I did want to know about her life because it wasn't mine.

Gerald returned with the mobile phone. He handed it to Simone and I watched as she used the tip of her fingers to touch the screen and search through a long list of numbers. There were no buttons and you just had to touch it to make it work. It was like something out of a film. I sat there thinking, *Wow, this really is the future*, expecting Doctor McCoy to walk through the door, hands on hips, saying, 'It's a phone, Jim, but not as we know it.'

'Right, found it.' Simone tapped the screen a few more times and placed the small phone to her ear. I stared at her, curious to see how she would conduct the conversation; more so how the person on the other end would hear her, given the mouthpiece was nowhere near her mouth.

She didn't talk into it like the *Star Trek* device I thought it was. Instead, she kept the phone in the same position throughout the conversation.

'Yes, okay, okay, yes, no, she doesn't want to go to the hospital.' She looked at me; my stomach churned again, then rumbled. I was hungry. 'Okay, yes, one moment.' She took the phone away from her ear. 'Babe, your doctor is on annual leave; he won't be in for another two weeks. You can see another doctor, but not until Monday.' I looked at Katie. I knew she was trying to send telepathic messages for me to go to the hospital. It wasn't an option. I shrugged my shoulders and nodded that it was okay. Any doctor would do, I didn't care. I was sure I would be back in 1992 before Monday anyway.

'Doctor Davies, five o'clock, then, yes, I'll bring her myself, okay, thank you.'

Simone placed the phone next to her and held my hand again. She didn't hang up. I continued to stare at the strange piece of technology, believing the receptionist was still on the other end listening. 'Are you okay with this, Nay?'

I nodded and whispered, 'Yeah, sure.'

Simone gave me a strange look. 'Why are you whispering?' she whispered.

I leaned in closer and looked at the device. 'She can still hear you.'

'Oh.' She laughed. 'It hangs up when you finish the call. It's automatic.'

'Wic-ked,' I said, still whispering. A world with this kind of technology reached beyond the realms of my imagination. The last time I had seen a mobile phone, it had been plastic, grey, and the size of a house brick with a black aerial sticking out of the top. Frankly, I thought men in wide-shouldered suits looked like right tossers walking down the street shouting into them.

'Are you okay, waiting four days to see a doctor, Nay?' Simone took the focus off the alien technology and back onto my brain.

'It's okay.' I smiled reassuringly and squeezed her hand. 'I'm okay. I'll be fine. It's most probably nothing, just a bad headache or something.'

My stomach rumbled again, alerting me to the fact that I hadn't eaten yet. *Does Adult Naomi not eat and is that why this body is so skinny?* I wondered.

Still, the only thing I could think of was pickled onions and cottage cheese.

Does the future still have them?

3
Déjà Vu

It's like I know
I have never met you before
but I feel like I have.
I think that's a soul memory;
you're remembering the life you've already seen,
the places you've already been.

L. E.

It was like déjà vu, but I couldn't stop it. I couldn't make it go away. I had this niggling feeling that I had seen everything – the people, the places and the things – before. But no matter how hard I tried, I just couldn't remember. And now I had to meet the child I knew belonged to Adult Naomi yet I couldn't remember giving birth to. Simone had taken the rest of the day off work and, not wanting to leave my side, decided to take me to the school herself. I wasn't ready to go back to the house of horrors I had woken up in, so Katie had invited us back to hers for dinner.

'What shall I say to him?' I asked Simone as we climbed

into a small bubble-shaped silver car with a strange-looking
number plate. I was well nervous.

'I don't know,' she replied. 'I mean, you could be okay and
go back to normal tomorrow and then we would scare him for
no reason. But . . .' She paused.

As grown-up as my sister had become, she still had that
same purse-lipped, narrow-eyed look when she was about to
say something sensitive. 'But . . . well, this could last longer
than a day.'

'It won't.'

'How do you know?'

'I just do.'

'But, Nay—' she protested

'No, Sim, I'm safe,* honest. I bet by the time I get to the
doctor's I'll be back to normal and I'll remember everything.'

I secretly hoped this wasn't the case, as I didn't really want
to remember anything about the past seventeen years. I had
only been in it a few hours but I was beginning to suspect that
the future wasn't turning out how I had imagined.

'I don't think we should tell him then,' Simone said quietly.

I agreed, and reckoned that with Simone and Katie's help, I
could pretend everything was okay for the night at least. Until
this awful feeling of déjà vu went and I would no longer be in
a city I didn't like the look of, living a life I just didn't get.

We arrived at the school and waited in the playground. A
couple of the mothers smiled at me, but none said hello or
came up to me, which Simone said was because it was a new
school and Leo usually went to something called After-School

---

* *Safe* – absolutely fine.

Club most days. I was kinda relieved but still really didn't want to be there.

What if Leo did suspect something? What would I do if I couldn't hide that I was fifteen from him?

A bell rang and shortly after, the doors burst open and a sea of children in royal-blue jumpers ran out, noisy and excited at the end of the day. My anxiety rose sharply and I wanted to chip*. Simone gripped on to my hand and squeezed it.

'Nay, you are going to be all right, okay?' she said. 'I trust you and Leo trusts you, and as scared as you are right now, wait until you see him. That fear will go, I promise.'

Leo was one of the last to exit the double doors, and he came out with his teacher, hands in his pockets, bag on his back. He was much taller than I expected, with the same complexion as me and a small afro of dark brown curls. I was speechless – there was this smaller version of me, but a boy. His eyes scanned the playground and, as soon as he spotted us, he gave us the most humongoid smile.

At that moment, something weird happened to me in the centre of my chest. I went all, like, slush puppies!** I breathed out. He was mine. There was no way I could say he wasn't my child. He walked like me and he definitely had that chipmunk-cheeked, dimpled, toothy grin that we were all cursed with. It was like looking at myself in one of those fun-house mirrors and seeing a three-foot version of me.

'Close your mouth, babe.' Simone reached over and pushed my jaw up. 'You'll catch a butterfly.'

---

* *Chip* – leave with great speed (nothing to do with potatoes).
** *Slush puppies* – feeling all kinds of mushiness for a person.

I smiled. 'Wow! I kid you not, Simone, he totally looks like me.'

'Oh yes,' she said, nodding, 'he's a mini you all right.'

'Wow, she had a boy,' I whispered.

He walked up to us, still smiling. I stood grinning at him.

'Hiya, mate.' Simone gave him a high five. 'Public displays of affection are a no-no to ten-year-olds,' she whispered to me out of the corner of her mouth. He high-fived her back, then looked at me expectantly. I had no clue what to do, so I followed Simone's lead and high-fived him too. He looked at me strangely, laughed, and placed his school bag into my hand instead. It was then that I figured mothers high-fiving their sons wasn't cool, but thought, *What's with the high-fiving anyway?*

'How was school?' Simone started to walk towards the school gates. Leo followed. I stood still, watching him as he tried to keep in step, telling her of the day's events. All of a sudden the mega-ness of what it would mean if I couldn't leave the future dawned on me. I had responsibility for a whole other person who, at that moment, had no clue that I didn't know him. As I watched him and my sister walk away, I started to feel something other than a desire to leave this future and be done with the whole nightmare. I started to feel that same chillness, like when I read the Irish blessing. Kind of, like, a hope that if I didn't fall asleep that night and wake up in 1992, that if I had to spend longer than I thought in 2008, as long as I knew him, as long as I hung around this cute, happy kid, then I would be all right. It was so weird to feel so stuck in between two places. I felt like I was being pushed away from the future and pulled towards it at the same time.

As if reading my thoughts, Leo turned around and shouted to me, 'Come on, Mum!'

Mum. Whoa! The word bounced against my head like a tennis ball in the drum of a dryer. 'Mum.' It tumbled out of my mouth. 'This is completely, totally, mega mental,' I said out loud and quickly made my way over to them, taking a hop, skip and a jump. He laughed at this and shook his head. I stopped and walked properly instead. By the time we had reached the car, he was happily chatting away about his day while I watched, fascinated by the way he spoke and the expressions on his face. I could have listened to him all day and night.

'What's for dinner, Mum?'

My smiled dropped and I looked at him in shock. *Dinner? Crap! Could I cook?*

Simone sensed my horror at the thought of having to feed this little person.

'It's okay, Leo, we're going to Katie's for dinner tonight,' she said as we climbed into the car.

'Yes!' Leo pumped his fist in jubilation.

'How was the rest of your day, mate?' Simone asked him.

'Yeah, good. Look, I swapped some new cards.' He pulled out a large pack of colourful cards.

I turned to him and said, 'Cool,' even though I had no clue what they were.

'What are they called again?' Simone asked him, probably for my benefit.

'My Yu-Gi-Oh! cards. Ben swapped four with me today and I got this one, look.' He pulled out a card and held it up to my face. It had a picture of a white dragon on it and the words 'Blue-Eyes White Dragon'. I tried to look really impressed.

'Nice one,' I said.

He giggled and sat back in the car. 'I can win the next battle now.'

'Wow, that's great that, mate,' Simone said to him. 'Do you have any homework?'

Oh crap, yeah. Mums ask about homework, don't they? I was finding hiding being fifteen from him harder than I thought.

He shook his head. 'Just gotta read my reading book later.'

'Okay, I'll listen to you read it before you go to bed,' Simone said. He seemed happy with this and carried on talking about his cards.

As I listened to him chat about school and his new friends, I realized that there were a lot of things I couldn't say because I didn't know or understand what he was talking about. This kinda made everything feel bogus again so I watched the streets go by instead. I started to feel excluded from a life I had no memory of. I zoned out of the conversation and closed my eyes.

The future.

We spent the rest of the evening at Katie's. She cooked dinner while Leo played with Dylan, Adam and Chloe. I didn't recognize them but they were more interested in Leo than me so pretending that I was an adult in front of them was easier. Alex, the oldest, was thirteen but he didn't want to be around any of us so stayed in his room until his dinner was ready. Every now and then we could hear him shouting from his room to someone. I thought he was having a party until Katie explained to me that he was talking to his friends through his computer.

I just stared at her for, like, ten minutes, trying to wrap my head around what she had said. I couldn't.

In the end, sat on the sofa, I started to feel chilled while Simone and Katie chatted and the children talked to each other. I thought their northern accents made them sound cute and cheeky, especially when they all started arguing about someone called Hannah Montana. Chloe loved her, but Dylan and Adam were teasing her about this Hannah, while Leo stuck up for Chloe.

Because I hadn't eaten all day I ate early with the children and watched on in amusement and awe as Leo's personality shone amongst his friends. I had to give Adult Naomi the most props*. He was an all-right kid, confident, bright, with a great sense of humour, which sometimes got a little silly when trying to impress the other children, who, I might add, found him hilarious. So did I. Simone gave us both a few stern words and serious looks, but he had the utmost respect for her and I shut up immediately, remembering I was supposed to be the adult. Making loud slurping noises while sucking on spaghetti until the sauce flew everywhere was not funny when you're thirty-two.

The children finished their dinner and went to play outside while I still had a half-full plate.

'I can't eat much. I don't have an appetite,' I said to Katie. 'I'm sorry.'

---

* *The most props* – to give someone the proper respect they deserve.

'It's okay, hun. You haven't had much of an appetite the last three months. You've lost a lot of weight.'

'Have I? Why?'

'You have just got over a bad case of tonsillitis – you couldn't swallow – and before that you had a stomach virus,' she said.

'Smegging hell!' No wonder I was skinny.

Simone and Katie seemed to be waiting for me to ask them about Adult Naomi's life and I managed to ignore the pain enough to ask a few questions. I wanted to know the basics at least before I went back to 1992, but not too much detail in case my head started to hurt again.

They told me that after moving around for a few years as a teenager, Adult Naomi had come looking for work and eventually settled in Manchester aged nineteen, and that she had been living in the city for thirteen years. So had Simone, who lived on the south side of Manchester. She said it was closer to her work.

'I work for a charity that provides educational and employment support for young people leaving foster care,' Simone told me. 'If they have children of their own, I work with social services and if they have mental health issues, I work with mental health workers, you know, give them extra support, help them find a job or get into education.'

'Cool,' I said.

'And I am a stay-at-home mum,' Katie added proudly. 'We met when we both used to live on the same street and our kids started to play together, do you remember? About five years ago now.'

I didn't remember. Simone continued to explain that where she lived was more culturally diverse and provided better access to the city. Adult Naomi, on the other hand, preferred the quieter, leafier Jewish suburbs in the north of the city. Okay. So that made sense to me: we had grown up in a small town, surrounded by lots of fields, woods and countryside. Even living in a city, they explained, Adult Naomi had gravitated to the greener parts. Having a partially deaf child meant she needed better services and schools for support.

'What? Hold up, wait a minute. Did you just say Leo is deaf?' I interrupted the conversation, stood up, and walked over to the patio doors to watch him. How had I missed this? He didn't use sign language. 'What d'ya mean, he's deaf?' I turned back to Simone. 'He doesn't talk like he's deaf.' Jeez, I felt awful; I hadn't even noticed.

She explained that Leo had been diagnosed with something called high frequency hearing loss when he was four and that without his hearing aids he could only hear vowel sounds and would have to read your lips to understand what you were saying. But with his hearing aids on and lip-reading he had a better chance of hearing you.

Although devastated at first, Adult Naomi had vowed to do her utmost to raise a healthy, well-rounded, confident child, and he now loved skateboarding, telling jokes and riding horses. She wouldn't allow him to use his inability to hear like everyone else as an excuse not to succeed in life.

'You're raising a bit of an extreme sports kid,' Simone laughed.

'Got no fear, that one,' Katie added. 'He's the bravest child I know.'

I stared out through the patio windows at Leo doing back and front flips on a large trampoline and laughing every time he landed. I felt a small hint of curiosity for Adult Naomi's life beginning to develop inside me. I wanted to know a bit more about Leo. I couldn't even remember giving birth to him. Simone explained that it had been a water birth. The relationship with his father? Katie just took a deep breath and blew out a gust of air. Her expression said, *You don't wanna go there*, but I learned that he was still a part of Leo's life. So I didn't ask any more about him because it made my head hurt too much. Besides, he wasn't fit Robert Harris so I didn't want to know. And just like my mum and my stepfather, if Leo's father wasn't around all the time, then I was beginning to guess that something was most probably wrong. I felt sick to my stomach.

I was still so not happy with what they were telling me. Adult Naomi had not been eating or sleeping properly for three months. Apparently, before the stomach virus and tonsillitis she had broken up with some French dude called Henri, which, according to Katie, had devastated her. She'd thought he was the love of her life. I nearly fell off my chair when she told me Adult Naomi had only spent two weekends with him in Paris. I mean, *hellooo*?! Just as bogus was the fact that Adult Naomi was unemployed, doing a degree she was struggling to finish, and living in a two-bedroom council house, driving a beaten-up Fiat Brava. What the smeg was going on? I couldn't help but think that this was *sooooo* not the way things were supposed to go. What had gone wrong?

'You keep a diary!' Katie exclaimed. 'You have done for as long as I have known you, actually.'

'I don't think you have ever stopped writing in it. Do you remember?' Simone asked.

I didn't. As far as I was concerned, at that point in time I had only been keeping a diary for five years. I needed somewhere to hide all my secrets and talk about all the stuff going on at school. Who I thought was fit and who was rank. What happened at Sara's party when we played Spin the Bottle. What the Mega Smegs were wearing on 'wear your own clothes day' at school and how they thought they were acting all stush.*

Apparently, Adult Naomi had continued writing them and had over twenty years' worth of diaries. I reckoned it was majorly sad that she still kept a diary. Hearing Katie and Simone tell me about Adult Naomi's life was easy – I didn't know her and it had nothing to do with me. I *so* didn't want to read her diary. I definitely didn't want to feel anything for this person whose future was completely alien to me. Besides, I was afraid of what I would find out.

Sack this, I thought. *Leo is cool and everything but he'll be fine with Simone and Katie until Adult Naomi comes back. I'm definitely going back to 1992 tonight.*

Katie sensed my unease. 'Well, you don't have to read them just yet; it might be a bit much for you.'

'Yeah,' I agreed. 'Too much, too soon.'

I realized I was too tired to take any more in and Simone said she would take me and Leo home. I didn't want to go at first. I kinda felt safe at Katie's, but had no choice. I had to get to sleep that night and get back to 1992.

Katie offered dinner again for the next day and Simone said she would leave work early to collect Leo from school. I was

---

* *Stush* – stuck up/like you smell of roses and nobody else does.

cool. By tomorrow Adult Naomi would be back in her body, her mind, her life, so I didn't have anything to worry about.

I got up from the table.

Don't think about it, Nay. Just go back to the house, find some pyjamas, climb into bed and sleep, I thought.

My body agreed. Yes, I was leaving the future. If I could find the doors in my dream again and walk through them, then I would get back to 1992 where none of this had happened and change things so that the future wouldn't turn out so bloody bogus.

After hugs and reassurances from Katie – I kinda liked her and felt a bit sad knowing I wouldn't see her again – we said our goodbyes to her family and Simone drove us back to the house.

'I'm tired, Mum,' Leo said as we climbed into the car. 'Do I have to read my reading book?'

'No, mate, it's okay. Just have a bath and go straight to bed,' Simone answered him.

'Yeah,' I said, 'you can read it tomorrow.'

He gave a sleepy smile and lay down in the back seat of the car. I remembered all of the times I had been left alone to look after the neighbours' kids and babies when my mum and her mates wanted to go to the pub. I deffo could look after him for just one night. He was a cool kid. He would be all right with me.

Ten minutes later, we pulled up outside the house. It was getting dark but I could see that it sat at the end of a narrow tree-lined lane with a large park nearby and a primary school down the road which wasn't Leo's school. Simone had told me rather matter-of-factly that the very bricks and mortar I had woken up in had provided Adult Naomi with a sanctuary at a time of her life when she had needed it the most.

And . . . ? I was so not impressed.

It had as much appeal as living in a caravan stuck at the edge of a cliff at the back end of nowhere during a wet and cold winter. I was embarrassed that she called it home. The broken gate, the unkempt gardens, the small windows and the old wooden door stared back at me mockingly. *Yes*, it said. *This is her house and she doesn't even own it and it's a big fat symbol of her complete failure at life.* I hung my head in shame, as my dreams of becoming very successful and living in a big house with at least six bedrooms, a pool and horses faded away. To see that seventeen years later I had not achieved what I was so convinced would rightfully be mine was rank bogusness. I was disappointed in Adult Naomi but I managed to push the ill-disguised disgust to the back of my mind. I was too young to entertain failure, and besides, this was not my life. I wasn't responsible.

We climbed out of the weird-shaped car and a cat came from behind the bushes and sat at the gate, licking her black paws.

'Hey, Sophia.' Leo bent down to stroke her; she purred furiously and rubbed her head against his hand.

'Is that ours?' I whispered to my sister so that Leo couldn't hear me. She nodded.

Leo walked through the gate and the cat followed him.

'I've got a cat?' I was mortified.

'Told you you'd end up an old lady with cats.' Simone laughed.

So not funny.

'I'm only joking, sis.' She slapped me on the back. 'Come on.'

Stepping around the yellow-eyed, meowing ball of black fur, I followed my sister and Leo into the house. This I couldn't deal with. Why the hell did she feel the need for a cat? I was so allergic to them and the only pets we had been allowed were two goldfish called Albie and Arthur that died after, like, a month 'cause we overfed them. I decided that somebody must have kidnapped the real her and replaced her with some Michaela Strachan clone from *The Really Wild Show*, all in love with animals and stuff.

Jeez.

Holding the door, I turned and looked at the cat. It meowed at me. I gave it the finger and slammed the door in its face, hoping it would disappear.

I was happy for Simone to put Leo to bed for the night. When he finished in his bath he came to the top of the stairs and shouted, 'Night, Mum.'

I went to the bottom of the stairs and shouted, 'Goodnight,' back to him.

He looked so cute with his shiny face and boy's blue pyjamas that I went all slush puppies again. The whole thing was getting a bit confusing for me but I said, 'See you in the morning, mate,' to him, hoping to sound a bit like Simone and a bit more like a mum. He smiled and went to his bedroom. I was curious to see the inside of the room I had stayed away from when I first woke up in the future, but I was afraid that if I liked it, I would like him even more and want to stay in the future. I couldn't; I had to leave. Adult Naomi had to come back.

I went into the kitchen instead. The kettle and toaster were a chrome silver that reminded me of something from *Blossom*. I looked again at the postcards and photographs lining the walls. Leo had been such a cute chubby baby. He and I seemed happy in them all, with big smiles, a radiance in our faces. It almost looked as if, at times, life was good. But I couldn't believe it. How dare Adult Naomi smile so happily given the way her life had turned out? And if she was so happy, why had she left?

It made no sense.

I pulled a postcard off the wall. It had the words '*Greetings from Rhodes*' on the front and a picture of blue waves kissing a white beach. I turned the card over; it was blank on the other side. I stuck it back on the wall and tore down another.

Atlanta! Wicked! I had made it.

The card read, '*Everything's peachy in Atlanta*' on the front, and the words were framed with pictures of peaches. Again this card was blank on the other side. Disappointed, I placed it back on the wall; I didn't bother to look at the ones from Portugal or New York. Had she actually visited these countries?

I walked back into the small wooden-floored living room, looked at the dark pink walls, and shuddered. What had possessed her to paint them that rank colour? There was a humongous TV in the corner and I marvelled at its massive rectangular-shaped shiny flat screenage. It looked like that huge TV on *Back to the Future II*. It was worlds away from the small cube-shaped television that I was used to. But how the smeg did you switch it on? There were no buttons. Had buttons been banned?

Simone found me staring at a tall wooden bookcase containing stuff that looked nothing like books.

'Leo okay?' I asked her.

'Yes, he's fine. He was tired,' she told me. 'It's been a long day. I told him you weren't feeling very well and that I was going to be around for a few days to take care of you both.'

'Cool.' I turned back to the bookcase. 'Err, what are these? There are loads of them.' I pulled a slim plastic case from the shelf. It had a picture of a red high-heeled shoe on the front.

'It's a DVD.' My sister joined me by the unit.

'What the frignacious is a DVD?' I flipped it over and saw film images on the back.

'It's a film on disc. Look.' She grabbed hold of a case from a shelf and opened it to reveal a round, thin, shiny silver object. I took it out of her hands and looked at my reflection in it.

'Is it a mirror as well?'

She burst out laughing and took another off the shelf. 'No, look, you play it on a DVD player.' She pointed to a slim silver machine underneath the television stand.

'Shut the front door! What happened to video?'

'Videos went out with *Record Breakers*, Nay.'

'There's no more *Record Breakers*? But Roy's still alive, right?'

Simone shook her head.

I couldn't believe that Roy was gone. I thought he would last forever. I asked her about TV. Apparently Simon and Trevor didn't swing their pants anymore, Phillip Schofield's hair had gone silver and he had swapped Gordon the Gopher for grown-up telly, and Andi Peters had retired Edd the Duck, and, well . . . was still Andi Peters. And Ant and Dec had left

Byker Grove and were searching for Britain's most talented celebrities in a jungle or sumthin'.

Like a magpie watching over its horde, I continued to marvel at the shiny silver object in my hand. There were numerous DVDs on the shelves. I looked through them, recognizing some of the titles like *Pretty in Pink* and *The Goonies*.

'But there are so many. Don't I do anything apart from watch these things? I mean, we watched films and stuff, but it looks as if I've turned into some kind of div film nerd.'

'No, Nay, this is cool. You've always loved films and there's nothing wrong with that. If you think about it, you've had to stay at home most of the time to take care of a child, so what better thing to do than watch movies?'

So far, *sooooo* offended, but instead I nodded, even though it seemed like such a waste of life. I thought of more interesting things I could do with my time than sit in front of a television all night, like, say, I don't know, build a multi-million-dollar empire *à la* J. R. Ewing.

I asked Simone why I had painted the living-room walls a spew-inducing salmon pink.

'You said you were going for a Tuscany vibe,' she answered.

I shuddered. I didn't get Adult Naomi's taste in decor, but the kitchen with its bright orange and yellow wasn't so bad.

'You were going for a Mexican feel,' she explained.

I followed her up to the bathroom and looked at the cream and beige walls, and the small shells and pictures of beaches lining the walls and shelves. 'Let me guess,' I said. 'I was going for the Blackpool feel.'

My sister laughed and then we walked into the bedroom

where this had all started, where I had woken up a few hours earlier, my life turned upside down. I looked at Simone for some futuristic-themed decorating explanation for the bare floorboards and grey plaster walls but she shrugged her shoulders.

'Don't know what happened here, babe. You started stripping, and well . . .'

She never finished, I thought. I looked around at the lovely bedroom furniture and wondered why Adult Naomi had not continued to make the place where she slept beautiful.

So not my problem. Knowing why meant going into *her* headspace, which I was still not willing to enter. But I reckoned the room would do, until I could leave the hamster cage of a house and go back to my lovely, warm, already decorated bedroom.

We made our way back downstairs and I noticed the other wooden units in the far corner of the living room. The larger one contained books and the smaller one held objects I did not recognize.

'I still read, then?' I let my eyes wander over the titles, everything ranging from Stephen King, which I recognized, to *Harry Potter*, which I didn't.

'Yep, still a bookworm. In fact, this is only a fifth of your collection.'

'What?' I spun around. There were at least two to three hundred books packed tightly on the shelves.

She nodded and pulled out a book called *Twilight*. I got a strange feeling when I looked at it.

'But Dad has the books stored in boxes because this house was too small for them.' Simone put the book back and noticed my stunned expression. 'It's okay. Your old house was much bigger than this, Nay.'

I slumped on the sofa, stared up at the books, then at my sister. 'And why am I not still living in this big house?'

She sat down next to me and put her arm around me. 'It's a long story, babe. I know you don't remember and I know it doesn't make sense, but it will. You gave the house up.'

'What? Why?' I rubbed my temples, trying to remember. I was beginning to feel sick again. Simone went into the kitchen to fetch me a drink. I grabbed the glass from her and took a large sip. Even the water tasted strange.

'Nay, listen, I promise you will remember everything and it will make sense to you. Just try not to force yourself to remember anything. We'll see the doctor on Monday and then at least we'll know what's wrong and what we can do about it. I'm sure he'll figure out how we can get your memory back.'

I nodded, and fake smiled; *I'm leaving tonight anyway*, I thought. My head was beginning to thump painfully and I was tired, very tired. I shoved over to make room for her and held on to her.

'Do you want me to stay? I can stay and leave for work in the morning,' she said.

'I know but, no, it's okay. I'm just gonna go to bed when you leave anyway.'

I didn't want to disrupt anyone's life any more than I already had and, seeing my sister's tired eyes, I knew I had to let her get back to some normality. She and Katie had been so calm all day. I had a strange feeling this wasn't the first time she had had to deal with something like this. Yeah, Simone might be an adult but she was still my little sister and I had to take care of her and make sure she was okay, and asking her to do any more than she had already done felt well selfish of me.

So I convinced her I would be fine to be left alone with Leo and that I was sure everything would go back to normal. She didn't want to go and I secretly didn't want her to leave me in what had to be *Nightmare* on frickin' *Elm Street*, but I told her to go home and come back the next day. Besides, Adult Naomi would wake up tomorrow, not me, and everything *would* go back to normal.

'Well, Leo basically wakes himself up for school, gets a quick wash, brushes his teeth and dresses himself. All you need to do is help him with his breakfast and give him this,' she said, handing me the *Star Trek* phone. 'He walks to school on his own now most of the time, so he'll call you when he gets to the school gates,' she continued, before showing me how to work the device. I was astounded at the fact that a ten-year-old boy had a mobile phone and dumbfounded at the size and capability of the small contraption. It was the same size as the one Adult Naomi had but you had to flip it open to make a call or answer it.

'Nay, can I ask you something?' Simone said.

I nodded, still trying to take everything in.

'Why do you keep saying "smeg"?'

I looked at her, puzzled. What a strange question. 'Smeg, smegging, smeghead?' I questioned *her* memory. '*It's cold outside. There's no kind of atmosphere. I'm all alone, more or less.*' I began to sing and click my fingers.

Perturbed, her eyes widened at my off-key attempts to sing the theme tune to my favourite programme.

'Lister? Rimmer? Cat?' Surely she hadn't forgotten. 'Oh my dayz, *Red Dwarf*!'

'That was your thing, Nay, not mine.'

'Was?'

'Yeah, sadly, smeg is no more. Craig Charles moved to *Coronation Street*.'

'What?' I laughed and then realized by my sister's expression that she was in fact telling the truth.

'It has been seventeen years, Nay.'

'Yeah,' I said, feeling dejected again. 'It really has.'

'But you can get it on DVD now, I think.'

'Cool,' I said. But it didn't feel cool; it felt well sad that *Red Dwarf* was no more.

My sister left for her own home, but not before she had been reassured countless times that I would be fine. She left me with all of her home and work numbers, and her mobile number. I took them, trying to figure out why people needed so many phone numbers. We agreed I would call her, no hesitation, if there was a problem.

I listened by his door to see if Leo was asleep. His room was quiet.

When I got into Adult Naomi's bed I curled my body up really small and squeezed my eyes tight shut. I thought if I concentrated enough, I would be able to somehow find Adult Naomi and return her to her body so that when I woke up the next day, I would be back in my own home and back in 1992.

My mind was a place of darkness; I couldn't hear or see a thing. Nothing or no one existed, not even the pain I had been feeling all day. My body was too exhausted even to hurt anymore.

Please, please, please, Adult Naomi, where the hell are you?

I pleaded with the darkness to stop hiding her, to stop hiding her memories and release me from my futuristic prison.

Then I saw it, a faint light in the distance. It felt like a dream; my eyes were closed, but I knew I wasn't quite asleep because I could still hear my own breathing.

I allowed myself to follow it and the more I focused on it, the bigger it got, until it got so close, it was undeniable. I was on a dark, deserted street, the only light provided by the orange glow of a street light. Behind me was a house. I called out and my voice echoed back to me, and then an eerie silence fell. *Where am I?* The sound of my breath faded and my body felt heavy; I drifted into a dream.

I turned around and found myself staring at a house, and as I did, a strange feeling crept over me. It was quiet, it was empty and the windows were dark, but I knew something. Then it dawned on me, the way the house made me feel. I had been here before. I couldn't remember, but it felt so familiar. I had that same feeling.

I had seen this house before.

It was déjà vu.

4

Window to the World

Sometimes the windows steam up
and you can't see what's outside
but then you take your finger
and make different shapes
on the glass inside;
that always makes me smile

N. S.

I had to push down every feeling inside of me to stop myself from screaming when I woke up the next morning. I was *still* in the same bed, *still* in the same room and *still* in the same house. I was *still* in the future. I tried to calm myself by counting the little bumps on the woodchip ceiling.

One, two, three, four, five . . . this isn't really happening to me . . . six, seven, eight, nine, ten . . . this sooooo can't be happening to me.

But it was and I couldn't stop it. I was majorly pissed off.

And then I remembered Leo.

He was already awake, sitting up in bed with a sleepy smile on his face.

'Good morning,' I said to him, sounding as happy as I could manage given how I felt.

'Mornin', Mum,' he said, halfway through a yawn, and climbed out of his bed.

I followed him around thinking he was cute bananas, watching him happily get himself ready for school, until he shoved me out of the bathroom for some privacy. He ate his cereal, packed his bag and put on his coat.

'Is it okay for me to skate later on, when I finish my homework?' he asked me as I opened the door for him.

'Err, yeah, sure.' I reckoned it would be okay.

'Yes!' He fist-pumped the air, kissed me goodbye, and was gone through the door quick time, leaving me standing there trying to style out* the daft grin on my face.

The sadness of still waking up in the future seemed to hide itself when Leo was around. He felt like my younger brother and I was kinda cool with playing the big sister while I was there. Adult Naomi's life was bogus, but I had to make sure he was okay. A few moments after he left I called him on his mobile. Telling him to have a kriss** day at school confused him, though. He called me lame and laughed at me.

I went back to Adult Naomi's bedroom, sat on her bed, and took a good look around, searching for any memories of her life or even the familiar house I had seen before I fell asleep. Nothing.

---

* *Style out* – pretend it's not really happening, when really it is.
** *Kriss* – really really (no seriously *really*) nice.

I decided to start with what I knew.

I know who I am, I told myself. *I'm Naomi Jacobs and I'm fifteen. I'm supposed to be revising for my smegging French exam, ugh! But I'm stuck in this frickin' place.*

I'm the daughter of my mum, Eve, and my dad, Art, who lives with his girlfriend Marlene in Liverpool – where I was born – and we visit them in the summer or at Christmas. I'm Simone's big sister and . . . okay, so, yeah, I don't, like, know everything, but I know life is a mix of the good, the bad and the downright bogus but I get it; well, I think I get it. I, like, wanna figure it out and do my own thing, make my own way in the world.

My mum says we left Liverpool when I was five because of the riots. I don't remember them but I kind of remember my step-dad, Joseph, moving in with us when I was about seven or eight. He has a trailer load of kids who come and stay for weekends or holidays and sometimes I think it's well cool having loads of stepbrothers and sisters, but other times it's bogus 'cause our house is so small and there are seven of them. One time, when I was twelve, I was so totally pissed off that there was no room, I slept in a sleeping bag in the bath. Joseph is mega, though; he gives me pocket money and plays the drums and always tells us these hard riddles that we never know the answers to. Apart from when he gives us loooonnnng lectures about the meaning of life, I think he's a safe stepdad.

Our house is in Wolverhampton, small town, small-minded people that talk about you all the time, and if they ain't got nothin' to say, they'll make it up. School's okay; some of my teachers are, like, total smegheads, but my friends are cool – I've got nuff love for my friends, even though most of them come from completely different backgrounds to me. I play sports at

school; favourites gotta be hockey of course . . . oh, and netball.
I really like, no, luurve eating chocolate. Deep down I am kinda
sensitive, and I do think a lot about stuff, but I can always make
the best out of any situation, can't I? Well, if you don't like me,
you can go and swing for all I care. Which I tell people to do on
a regs,* and the things I don't wanna share with peeps I share
with my diary.

The diaries!

I got off the bed and looked around the room. It didn't take
me long to find the diaries packed away in a cardboard box
under the bed. I pulled it out. It was full of books of different
sizes and colours. Some had patterns on the front; others were
plain. Some were bound in leather; others hardback.

My head started to pound again.

No, not yet.

I pushed the box back under the bed and carried on trying to remember what I knew about myself. This somehow
stopped the thumping pain.

From what Katie and Simone had told me the night before,
I figured Adult Naomi's life was the complete opposite of how
I thought it should have turned out. It felt like I was watching
her life standing on the other side of a window.

In the future she was still the daughter of Eve and Art, but
Art had had another child, a boy called JJ who was eighteen
years younger than she was. Eve was miles away and I figured
out Adult Naomi wasn't speaking to her. I didn't know why
and I didn't want to know. Besides, Simone and Katie seemed
to go quiet or change the subject every time I said her name.

---

* *Regs* – on a regular basis.

I was still Simone's big sister, but of course the biggest thing was Adult Naomi actually having a son, which I didn't quite get. On the one hand, I didn't understand her decision to have a child in the first place, and on the other, to do it and not marry the guy. Okay, Art and Eve never married, but surely Adult Naomi would if she wanted to settle down and have a kid. Didn't she, like, *want* a husband?

I kinda wanted to meet Leo's father, but at the same time, didn't want to know who Adult Naomi had chosen. There had to be a reason she wasn't with him and I got the sense from Katie and Simone's reactions that it wasn't a good reason.

What I totally didn't get was that she was doing a degree in psychology of all things. I mean, come on, why would she want to sit and figure out people's problems for a living? So she could graduate, she had to sit four final exams and was trying to revise before she disappeared. Is this why she disappeared? She didn't want to take her smegging exams!

I wanted to write. Or be a news journalist and see the world. Did the fact that she'd had a child change all of that? I didn't really know about Adult Naomi's behaviour, or the way she felt about stuff, but I figured her life couldn't have been that great, considering she smoked cigarettes, drank way too much coffee, and hardly slept.

What happened to you, Adult Naomi?

No, I thought. *What happens to me? Do I pass my exams? Does Robert Harris find out if I fancy him? Does Simone eventually stop using my hair gel? Do I have anything to do with the way the future has turned out?*

*

Katie phoned me when she got back from taking her kids to school to see if I was okay. I told her I was and that Leo was cool. She reminded me that if I needed her I only had to call her and she would come around straight away. She seemed to be a good friend to Adult Naomi and I was glad she was in her life.

Simone got the afternoon off work and came home to find me curled up on the sofa staring at the flat screenage, disturbed on some other totally mental level. What the hell had happened to TV?

'Sim, they all look like cartoons.' I was hypnotized. Technicoloured faces stared back at me, features animated to within an inch of their life, with these sharp, intense rainbow colours that somehow highlighted each pore, each line, each wrinkle, each crease of their skin. I could see every tiny movement, every step, every wave of an arm or expression on a face. It was like that moment when Dorothy opens the door of her sepia-toned fallen house and reveals an intensely hued kaleidoscopic Oz on the other side.

Simone sat next to me. I stared at her clothes: washed-out denim jeans and a thick blue hoodie with the words 'Abercrombie and Fitch' on it. Wasn't Abercrombie a street name in Liverpool? And who was Fitch? I shrugged it off; maybe it was the new fashion, to wear expensive-looking jumpers named after random streets. What had happened to Fruit of the Loom? Was there still Benetton? What about LA Gear?

'It's digital TV, babe.' She took the remote from my hand.

I flicked over to a channel actually called 'Reality TV' and watched as it advertised reruns of a show called *I'm a Celebrity . . . Get Me out of Here!*

'Please tell me, what the Gaddafi is this all about?' I said.

'No memories yet?' asked Simone.

I shook my head, mesmerized by the scenes playing out in front of me of unknown adults in goggles eating insects and trying not to throw up.

'Why are they doing this?' I asked her.

'Because they're sad, and they used to be famous and now they're not,' Simone replied.

'*This* makes them famous again?'

'Yeah. Well, only the winner. The rest just leave with a fat cheque in their pockets. They say it's for charity, though,' she finished.

I looked back at the TV. 'Duh, so run a marathon then! What has happened to TV, man? Where are, like, all the real programmes? Is there still Channel 4?'

'Yeah, but they have *Big Brother*,' she replied.

My only reference to the term 'Big Brother' was from an Orwell book called *1984* that I'd read when I was thirteen. My dad had let me watch the John Hurt film, which had led to me reading the book. It was unsettling on many levels. Did I even want to know what the future version entailed?

As I sat and listened to her, my mind became totally disturbed. I was shocked to hear how people with no talent became rich and famous overnight by actually doing nothing other than allowing millions of people to watch them. My fear of this unknown phenomenon translated into hostility and I deemed it sick, bordering on the weird. I couldn't believe it when she told me Adult Naomi had actually enjoyed watching *Big Brother* and had invested time and energy into following it. No wonder she hadn't built her empire! She was watching this pants.

I couldn't handle any more information. I jumped up from the sofa and pressed the off button, my hands trembling. 'This is madness, total mental madness,' I said. 'I don't get it.'

Concerned at my indignation, Simone suggested I get dressed and she take me food shopping.

'Your cupboards are bare,' she said, grabbing a black hand-bag from the side of the sofa. 'You're going to need some money from the cashpoint.'

'Money?' I was mystified. 'I have money? Where from? I don't bloody work.'

'Now, Nay, don't freak out, okay . . .' She held up her hands.

'What?' I said slowly, unsure if I wanted to hear what she was about to tell me. Although I knew it couldn't top the 'Adult Naomi didn't even own the crappy house she lived in' fact.

'Well, you have basically been living off a student loan for the past few years. You have some savings, but your weekly costs are covered by income support,' Simone stated.

'Income what?'

'It's a weekly payment you get from the government to help with the cost of living—'

'From the government?' I jumped up, interrupting her explanation. 'I'm a single mother on the *sosh*?*'

'Nay, calm down.' She lowered her hands.

'Calm down! Calm frickin' down! Are you smegging *serious*, Simone? I'm on social security? Oh God, this is worse

---

* *Sosh* – pronounced *So-shhh*. The word for social security or welfare as it's known today.

than I imagined.' I burst into tears and, swinging my arms around, I flung myself down onto the sofa.

Living in Manchester, I could just about deal with. Having a son, I was managing to get my head around. Being single wasn't a total surprise. But living a life in which I was doing a degree I would never use and taking weekly government handouts to survive brought on a whole other level of shame and anger at Adult Naomi.

I was cracking. The hot tears felt acidic as they stung my face. Simone put her arm around my shoulder.

'Nay, listen to me, you've got to stop reacting like this. You're going to make yourself ill. You've only been on this money since you lived in this house. You have worked every single day of your life since you were sixteen.'

I gulped back the taste of bile in my throat. 'I have?'

'Yes. You have even run three businesses successfully; two of them were your own.'

'Have I?'

She nodded. 'One was a friend's haulage company you helped run when you were twenty-one, when Leo was first born, and the other two, you were a teacher and therapist.'

'So what happened, Sim?'

Being told Adult Naomi had run three businesses seemed to spark something inside me. I felt like an artist restoring the colours on a faded canvas and in those last few moments I had somehow become sensitive to the details of her life. For the first time since I had woken up in the future, I really wanted to know what had happened. Even as a little kid I had possessed an 'entrepreneurial spirit'. My mum reckoned it was because when I was a baby, I always seemed to attract money, no matter where I went or who I met. I was like a pudgy pirate in Pampers – someone always crossed my palm with silver. Seeing quite a lucrative opportunity here, when Eve and Art had no money for bread and cigs, they would dress me in my finest and take me down the pub. People would coo over how gorgeous a baby I was and dip in their pockets. The drunker they were, the more they gave. And as I grew older, I got a feel for money. I liked getting it and having it and spending it. So I developed a talent for selling. My wares were anything from shrunken crisp-packet badges to sweets from my own tuck shop. If I could sell it, I would. School was my market and I was *The Fresh Princess of Belle Queenswood Comprehensive* ready to make my fortune.

Had Adult Naomi lost that entrepreneurial spirit?

Simone tried to explain. 'Nay, it's a long and complicated story, and if I tell you, you will try and remember and your head might start hurting again.'

As if on cue, a sharp pain stabbed at the back of my skull. I held on to my head and winced.

'Do you want a painkiller?' She stood up. 'Or a drink?'

I thought about what my sister had just said. I couldn't deny any longer the need to know who Adult Naomi was and the life she had created for herself. I made a solemn promise to myself that if by Monday I was still stuck in the future, then I was going to find out just exactly what had happened to her.

Simone returned from the kitchen with a glass of water and a small white pill.

'Listen, at least you haven't given Jeremy Kyle a call yet, so all hope is not lost, okay?' She smiled reassuringly at me.

'Who the frick is Jeremy Kyle?'

'He's like Jerry Springer, but British and angry, and a bit of a dick really.'

'Oh God. My life is over.' I placed the painkiller on my tongue, drank the water in one big gulp and slammed the glass down on the bookshelf next to the sofa several times. It sounded like a judge slamming a gavel, calling order to a chaotic court.

'This cannot be real, this cannot be my life,' I said.

I thought of Katie and her suggestion I should go to hospital. I felt like I should go, but there was something stopping me.

I needed to change the subject. 'Did you say there isn't any food?' I asked Simone.

'Well, there is, but you need bits – milk and stuff.'

'Let's go shopping then.' I stood up and straightened my crumpled pyjamas as if this act would somehow smooth out my thoughts. 'I'll have a quick bath and get dressed.'

'Okay.' My sister picked up the remote. 'I'll just watch a bit of MTV while you do.'

I turned to see an image of half-naked girls simulating sex moves, rubbing their bodies against each other and gyrating suggestively over a rapper reclining in a chair. I shuddered. Oh, it was all so wrong, so, so wrong. What else was I going to discover about the planet? About this life? And more importantly, how was my fifteen-year-old mind going to cope?

Fighting my curiosity was exhausting me. On the one hand, I wanted an explanation before I left, but on the other, I was afraid to know too much in case it meant that I would remain in the future. It worried me that I might find out too much about Adult Naomi, like her, get attached and not be able to leave her world behind.

As I ran the bath I thought that maybe Adult Naomi was in that house, the one I had seen in my mind before I'd fallen asleep. Maybe I could somehow get in through a window and look for her. Maybe I could find her, make her return and I could get out of the future.

In the meantime, the easiest choice was to blank everything as much as I could. Whatever hurt the least. I climbed into the bath and agreed with myself that, yes, maybe it was better to ignore that house and look to others to take over. The problem was that the only three people who could do this for me were my sister, Katie – a woman who had known Adult Naomi for five years – and a ten-year-old boy. On the other hand, I couldn't help but feel that if I wanted to get out of the future, the house was the only way. And if I wanted to know more, I would have to venture further out into Adult Naomi's world.

As I got dressed, I suddenly thought, *What if I can't ever leave the future? What if I'm stuck here and I've got no way of getting home? What if Adult Naomi doesn't come back?*

In the wardrobe mirror I caught sight of my aged face. In spite of the dark circles around my eyes, the spots and the boobs that no longer defied gravity, I still cared about the body in which I had awoken. The thought of possibly having a brain tumour was the stuff of nightmares, and I didn't want to put this body at risk or through any unnecessary harm. I wondered what could be hiding inside of me so terrible that could cause brain damage. What was so bad that Adult Naomi had had to leave and take seventeen years with her?

If I was still here the next day and the day after that, I would have no choice. I would have to get to know the parts of Adult Naomi's life I had been ignoring.

But first it was time for me to venture out into this strange and unfamiliar world with my sister.

Out into the future.

5

Global Warning

An eye for an eye
will make the whole world
blind.

Mahatma Gandhi

The future is now called the twenty-first century and it's kinda, like, a bit freaky, like *Freaky Friday* – freaky in the way that you know it belongs but it doesn't quite fit.

The future has:
laptops
and MacBooks
and PCs
and desktops
and USB sticks
and touch-screen phones
and iPods
and the Internet
and Google
and Facebook

and YouTube

and reams and reams and reams of information.

Simone explained all this to me on the way to the shops. My brain was smacked speechless.

I mean, we had computers at school, with massive keyboards and small black-screened monitors, and when you typed the letters were orange. If you were Mulder and Scully, you had one of those newfangled computers with a bright blue screen and white letters that you could type your X-files into. The computer Art bought us a couple of Christmases ago was a Commodore 64 and the program played on a tape machine. And Joseph got us one of those new front-loader video players when Mum threw out the top-loader Betamax. But TV kinda takes the piss out of the new car phone/mobile phone idea. They're for those suited, 'Loadsa Money'-type banker gits who drive red sports cars and carry Filofaxes.

The future also has:

chip

and pin.

It totally blew my brain when my sister and I stood in front of the cashpoint machine while she showed me how to use my 'debit' card. I remembered cashpoint machines but these were, like, *sooooo* different. I stood there, smegged to silence by the colour screen and mini camera watching me like a suspicious eye.

Like Katie's telephone number, Simone and I guessed the four-digit number going around in my head was in fact attached to the card. I was confused. Why could I remember numbers?

Simone parked outside a humongous Tesco.

'Whoa!' I stopped and stared at it. 'I thought we were only popping out for bread and milk?'

She turned the engine off and climbed out.

'Where are the shops?' I asked her, following.

'There aren't that many local shops anymore; the big supermarket chains have forced most of them out of business and pretty much taken over everything.'

As we walked through the automatic doors, I noticed a large sign at the entrance that told the shopper that it was an 'eco-friendly' store.

Simone continued to explain to me that Wal-Mart had taken over Asda Dales and dropped the Dales, Tesco now offered everything from petrol to credit cards, and Netto, Lidl and Aldi were new and popular cheaper supermarkets from Europe.

As we walked through the aisles of this gigantic place, my senses were slapped silly by the smell of freshly brewed coffee, baked bread and roasting chickens. My stomach rumbled loudly and I felt the sudden need to buy as much food as I possibly could. I followed my sister around and couldn't believe the variety of foods on offer – Kosher food for the Jews, Halal meat for the Muslims, Caribbean spices for the Caribbeans, Polish food for the Poles, and even tacos for those with a desire for Mexican food. There was gluten free, sugar free, wheat free, dairy free. The choice was endless. They didn't have the familiar orange and white labels of Happy Shopper, which was the cheapest brand on the corner shop shelves when I was a kid.

And what was this 'organic' food everywhere? Simone explained what it meant and I was baffled why people would choose to buy food full of chemicals anyway. She said that some people didn't have a choice, that there was now something called 'genetically modified' to deal with the growing demand for food and the increasing world population. My brain so couldn't deal. I felt like a small child wandering up and down the aisles of Willy Wonka's Chocolate Factory staring in awe and wonder at the limitless stuff available. How did you make a choice?

'Is there anything you want, sis?' Simone stopped, pivoted, and headed back up the dairy aisle. I was staring at rice milk, trying to figure out how you got milk from rice.

'Erm, cottage cheese.' I put the rice carton back on the shelf. 'Oh, and pickled onions.'

Simone stopped and turned to me.

'You don't eat dairy, especially not cottage cheese.' She pushed the trolley on.

'I don't eat dairy? What? Like, I don't drink milk?'

'Nope, nor cheese or ice cream. Well, sometimes you allow yourself ice cream, but not much because it runs your stomach.'

I burst out laughing. 'Runs it where?' I watched as she put the 'dairy-free' butter into the trolley. 'Are you squerious?*'

'Yep, you don't eat dairy or pickled onions. I haven't seen you eat those since . . .'

She paused and looked at me intently.

'What? Since when?'

---

* *Squerious* – meaning square and serious. Someone who fails to think 'outside the box', who is out of touch or behind the times, and takes things rather seriously (as if they were quite proud). Used extensively to express shock in the 1992 film *Wayne's World*.

'Since you were fifteen.'

I rolled my eyes at the yogurt pots and followed her as she set off again.

'What? Why does it make me ill? What happened?'

'You turned vegan.' She manoeuvred the trolley round me. I was glued to the floor, staring into the frozen-food space, confused. A vegan? I don't, like, eat anything except vegetables?

The only vegans I had ever known were Pippa and Robin, a couple of long-haired hippies who used to live a few doors away from us. They and their four white-blond-haired rosy-cheeked kids were vegans and they were, like, always skinny and always happy. I was chubby and miserable, but thought they were weird and cool. I used to sit with Pippa outside their house on summer nights while the children played barefoot on the street and she sang to herself while making daisy chains and beaded necklaces.

Robin loved music and taught me the first three chords of the James Bond 007 theme tune on his battered guitar. Before I had to go home, Robin would bring out his small metal pan pipe and Pippa would dance around in her long flowing skirts and tie-dyed tops, encouraging me to dance with her. I used to wish I were the fifth child in their little hippie, vegan, barefoot life. I was totally morosed out when they left for a five-bedroom house in the posh part of town, and confused at how two people who didn't work, who sat on cushions instead of sofas, could afford such a big place. And then one day, a neighbour told me it wasn't the meat-free, vegetable-only diet that made them so laid-back and happy; it was the amount of magic mushrooms they ate and the mounds of weed they smoked.

Clearly, Adult Naomi was no hippie; she wore skinny Morrissey-type jeans, Ugly boots and loose-fitting jumpers, which were supposed to be dresses. I didn't feel the need to play pan pipes or make daisy chains and yet here I was, standing in the middle of this ginormous food mecca, trying to get my head around the apparent crapation of my taste buds.

Coffee? No milk? Ugh! The thought made want to blow many serious chunks all over the Formica-tiled floor. No, I wanted cottage cheese and pickled onions and no one was gonna get in my way. Eventually we found the largest tub of cottage cheese and an even larger jar of pickled onions. I wondered why everything had grown to, like, three times its size.

Cottage cheese and pickled onions were all I ever ate. Well, that and jacket potatoes and salad, low-fat crisps and bananas. By thirteen, I was fat and though people said I 'carried it well' and that I didn't look 'that heavy', compared to all of my many skinny friends I felt big and clumsy. And then Sister Sugar Puff Teeth (the school nurse; she had bad teeth) told me that I had to lose weight. I cried to my dad on the phone and he put me on a thousand-calorie-a-day diet. Then I got, like, totally obsessed with calories and realized that cottage cheese and pickled onions – the strongest tasting vegetable that could prop up the tasteless cheese – were my best friends. But my stomach couldn't handle it so I became kinda part-time bulimic, binging on a regs, and then throwing it all up. It's just *tooooo* hard to function on celery and crackers.

According to Simone this lasted on and off – mostly on – until I turned eighteen and discovered something called amphetamines. I decided I didn't want to know what the Gaddafi they were so asked her more about being vegan.

She explained to me how, when Adult Naomi was twenty-four and she was studying Chinese Medicine at university, she decided to change her diet to vegan and did a lot of yoga. Apparently, her chickpea burgers were to die for and she was quite happy living the kelp and brown rice lifestyle.

'Well . . . what happened then?' I was fascinated and repulsed all at the same time.

'You quit uni, started smoking weed again, ate red meat, and decided to be a psychologist.' Simone picked up some bin bags and threw them in the trolley.

The Linda McCartney (not just Paul's wife but creator of meat-free food) soya sausages (sausages from a bean?) and rice milk lifestyle sounded well better than a steak-eating, stoned psychologist.

Simone did her best to buy as many things as she thought Leo and I would eat while I followed her, cast under the supermarket spell. It went something like this: 'Buy one, get one free, no, two for the price of one; better still, three for the price of two, or how about save £s and double up your points.' *Points?* You were rewarded for shopping?

I lost count of the amount of cameras watching us. What were they watching anyway? Surely people would be too afraid to rob anything; you'd have to run a marathon to get to the door with your stuff. Wasn't it only a matter of time before some government-approved robot would jump out of the eco-friendly fridge and rugby tackle you to the ground?

My senses seriously smegged into a shopping stupor. I stood in a daze, watching my sister interact with a different kind of computer, which told her to place her items in the bagging area, and asked which method of payment she was using.

No shopkeeper, no sales assistant, except for a woman who stood at the head of the machines and ran to the rescue if your items wouldn't scan.

Scan?

Simone told me that the barcode had taken over the shopping experience and was supposed to make everything much more 'convenient'.

Disturbed beyond reality, by the time we'd reached the car, I realized there was something missing. It was the familiarity of the local shops, the friendliness of the staff that you got to know during your weekly shop. The megastore was cold and clinical, with *way* too much choice. And yet there was something inside me that made me feel that if I kept going back, I would one day have the friendly experience I had just now left without. Was this how everyone who had swapped the local shop for the supermarket felt? Were they waiting to visit enough times so that eventually someone would recognize them, stop, and chat with them? Like a *Cheers* for lonely customers.

Where everybody knows your name.

I was missing home – the local village where everyone knew my name, or rather my mum's, and the smaller shops you left with a smile or a clip round the ear if you tried to nick something. My head was starting to hurt. I needed another painkiller as my shopping expedition had only left me with more questions. I also had a sudden urge to eat a Marathon and read a newspaper.

'Oh, why didn't you say? We could have got you one from Tesco's.' Simone slowed the car down. 'Shall we go back?'

'No, I don't want one from there. I want one from a news-paper shop.'

'Erm, right, okay.' She pulled out of the large car park. 'I think there is one in the village.'

I craved some small-town reality. If I could get just a small dose, maybe it would make the thumping pain go away.

Minutes later, Simone pulled into a much smaller car park behind a bank. On the opposite side was a row of shops including a newsagent's. I smiled triumphantly and jumped out of the car, passing a library and a chemist on my way. I could understand why Adult Naomi had chosen to live here. It reminded me of home and instantly, as if by some memory magic, the pain tearing through my skull subsided. I walked into the shop, a psychedelic purple and silver note in my hand, and bought a few newspapers and as many magazines as it could afford, which was, like, *four*.

I also asked the guy for a Marathon. He looked confused, then laughed and pointed at a Snickers. As I left the shop, I couldn't help it any longer. I had to get to know about the world I found myself in, here and now. In the supermarket, Simone had started to tell me about people's attempts to live life in an eco-friendly way, that because they were wearing out the planet, everyone was now recycling, reusing, geneti-cally modifying and saving energy. But what the smeg was a carbon footprint or global warming? Was that the same as the greenhouse effect we were told about at school? And what was this thing called the Internet?

I had woken up in the future and as I walked back to the car, I figured I should fill my mind with as much information about the world as possible before I left. It was a better option to filling it with Adult Naomi's memories and maybe it could help in understanding why she had left.

I was on a mish. I was going to go *global*.

By the time we had finished shopping, Simone needed to collect Leo from school; we ate at Katie's, and went back home early.

They let me pick the film, so we sat down to watch *Back to the Future* on UKTV Gold. I felt like I was Marty himself, except there was no Doc, and no help to guide me through the maze of a confusing future or a mysterious past.

After another night filled with tossing and turning and strange dreams, I woke up to Simone snoring next to me and Leo standing by my bed, asking if he could have a sausage sandwich. His wide, dimple-cheeked smile quickly washed away any terror that had piggybacked itself from my sleep and I figured I could work the grill out to make him breakfast.

It wasn't long before we were sitting on the sofa together, eating tomato-ketchup-laden 'chicken sausage' (?) sandwiches while we watched Saturday-morning programmes on the Disney Channel. Even though I couldn't remember anything about him, I liked being around and spending time with Leo. Every fear I had about myself, the world or this strange life seemed to disappear the moment he looked at me with his gorgeous brown eyes. On hearing his cute laugh, my confused existence became as clear as it could be. It made me feel real. Like I belonged. It was kinda strange, but as I watched him giggle at the slapstick programme about twin boys living in a hotel with a single mother, I wondered whether this was what Adult Naomi felt like around him. Protective and proud.

Kinda like a big sister. And hey, it seemed like single mother-
hood wasn't as bad as I'd first thought. Well, Disney didn't
think so.

The smell of cooked sausages woke Simone up. Once we
finished our breakfast, she suggested we go out for the day,
maybe to her house, and then for a walk. Leo was happy –
apparently he had friends in the gated community where she
lived – but I *sooooo* did not want to leave the house. I was still
digesting everything that I had experienced in the futuristic
supermarket and needed time to chill, absorb it all.

My ignorance was making me feel exposed, vulnerable, as
if I should know everything about the world, but didn't, so
was, like, really stupid. I wondered if Adult Naomi felt like
that or if it was just me. So I faked extreme head sensitivity
and told Simone I wanted to rest for the day. Besides, I still
had all of the newspapers and magazines to get through and
needed to know more about the world before I ventured back
into it. Simone and Leo left. I went back to bed and curled up
under the duvet to indulge in my papered realm.

The magazines fascinated and horrified me. I was used to
Just Seventeen and *Smash Hits*, looking at pictures of Take
That and NKOTB, doing the girly quizzes about boys – what
they think, how to get one, and how to keep one once you
have one – getting tips from supermodels Naomi Campbell or
Linda Evangelista on how to get fuller lips. If my friends and I
wanted a gossipy glossy, we'd buy *More* and sit in the back of
French class curling each other's eyelashes and taking the piss
out of the 'Position of the Week' section. Fast forward seventeen years and *More* just seemed to have . . . more. More men,
more make-up, more fashion, more sex, more, more, more.

Cosmo followed, as did *Vogue* and *Marie Claire*. I flipped from page to page, reading shocking true stories of women from around the world who were suffering from unimaginable oppression and poverty, only to flip over the page and see a model draped all over a Gucci bag. Adverts for petrol-guzzling cars sat next to articles about ice caps melting and severe weather disasters and saving the polar bears. I was freaking out. These magazines were contradictory, schizophrenic, masochistic publications that flaunted extreme wealth on the one hand, yet exploited poverty on the other.

The fashion was as strange as the Ugly boots. Embellishment! Everything was 'embellished': bags, shoes, jackets, all studded with metallic gold and silver studs. The dress of the season was 'bandage'. Exsqueese me? Didn't that usually happen if you'd hurt yourself?

But the thing that freaked me out the most was page after page of perfect-looking people. I mean, come on, where were the freckles, spots, blemishes? And what had happened to real bodies? What was with the size zero?

Was this for real? Did people, like, really wanna be, like, NO SIZE? I mean, AT ALL? As if! 'Nobody looks like this in real life,' I said out loud. This is impossible! WHAT THE SMEG HAS HAPPENED?

This was beyond absurd. My brain was having a total spaz attack! I threw down the magazines in disgust. I felt patronized and suddenly very inadequate, like when Mr Benson, headmaster of my school, had told me off for telling my typing teacher to go and throw her knickers in the air and see how time flies while I was walking out of my exam. This feeling was supposed to end with school, but something told me Adult Naomi and half the female population on the planet had become accustomed to it. It was inevitable if they read these types of magazines. How could anyone live up to what they saw in those pages? The flawless skin, the skinny bodies, the exclusive get-yourself-into-debt-for-fashion store card, the celebrity diet, and then the fatty recipes on the next page. The whole thing about how wine is bad for you, chocolate is good, no, wine is full of antioxidants (huh?) and chocolate is bad; exercise should be done two times, no, three times, no, four times a week, for ten minutes, no twenty, no, no less than thirty; eat berries and lose weight (duh), no, eat burgers and lose weight (*duh*).

Relationships – what he's thinking; who cares what he's thinking? But you're an independent woman and you don't need a man; still, you can find The One before you're thirty. Sex is good, but it can kill you (?). Sex is bad and you'll go to hell or join a cult and give up your life to the Prophet.

The whole lifestyle dumping truck of 'you're not good enough no matter what you do' shebang!

I mean, my fifteen-year-old mind knew it was pointless chasing after something that was never going to happen, hence walking out of the exam (who wants to type for a career anyway? It wasn't 1950). And yet I had an eerie sensation that I wasn't alone in the weird sense of lack I felt after reading those magazines, the same way I had felt after our supermarket sweep.

Something was missing.

Kinda like that feeling when someone tells you a joke, but you're stuck in a five-second delay before you get the punchline? Kinda like that.

I turned to the newspapers, starting with the red tops. The April weather was going to be full of cloud and rain. There was still a Page Three girl proudly showing off her boobs, no sign of a pencil case. People were still dying in the most heinous ways and a young African-American senator was running to be president of America and was ahead in the polls.

Hold up, wait a minute! Did I read right? I flipped over the page to see if the next page contained some crap journalist's idea of Joke of the Month, but found no such thing. For real, a black man was hoping to take up residence in the White House. People were actually positive he had a chance of winning.

I picked up the mobile phone and, concentrating hard, remembered Simone's demonstration of how to call her.

'Hiya, babe,' she answered, sounding upbeat. 'You okay?'

'What? Oh yes, totally, yeah, I'm fine. But sis, is it real, that, like, is there, like, gonna be a black president of America?'

'What? Erm, yeah, well, that's what they reckon if Obama wins.'

'Shut the front door! No. Way. Jose!' I was stunned.

'Serious, this is big stuff, and after the last president, America needs hope; the whole bloody planet does.'

'Why, what happened?' I so wanted to know.

'Why don't you Google it?'

She reminded me that Leo had shown me how to use the computer the night before. Apart from the odd strange look and question of 'Don't you remember this?' he had seemed to accept the excuse that I was helping him practise for senior school. To this, he replied that it was now called 'high school' and rolled his eyes. I stuck my tongue out at him and then remembered I was supposed to be a mum and straightened my face.

Why was the UK Americanizing everything? First high fives, then everyone started using the word 'lame', then super-sized food, and now schools have grades not years. *Is this what happens when you go global?* I wondered.

I hung up the mobile on my sister and followed the steps to access Google. Fascinated by its ability to produce endless information at the touch of a button, I decided whoever invented the Internet was top frickin' bananas. I wanted to venture into the unknown terrain of cyberspace.

As far as my world went, the closest I got to politics was *Spitting Image*, those large rubber puppets of MPs or pop and film stars. Most of the political jokes were beyond me, but I just loved it when they did Michael Jackson's heliumed voice, and I always creased up laughing at the size of Mick Jagger's exaggerated lips. In 1992, Bill Clinton was running for the American presidency; John Major had been elected Prime Minister here and was penned the dullest politician to ever walk the planet until he started attacking single mums, saying they were raising a generation of sociopaths and criminals. George Bush Sr and his band of 'Coalition Forces' had not long kicked Saddam's arse out of Kuwait and back to Iraq. None of this really affected me; if I ever caught *Spitting Image*, the rebel leader they took the piss out of was Colonel Gaddafi who was reportedly behind the murder of a British police officer outside of the Libyan Embassy and the Lockerbie bombing. In the future, I suddenly wanted to know exactly what had happened since.

My sister had told me to Google three words: George

Bush Jr. I did just that and was absolutely and utterly horrified as I read about the horrors of 9/11 and 7/7. It took me most of the day and I needed to take a few breaks in between but I spent hours reading article after article about the War on Terror.

Tears flowed heavily down my face as I read of the lives lost and the families devastated by the attacks. This search for 'weapons of mass destruction' had led to a war that was still raging, and to websites of endless conspiracy theories about the whole administration. They were after oil, and the Twin Towers was a set-up by the American government themselves; George Jr was just going after Saddam for revenge (or to impress his dad). Many protested about the war all over the world, from the Oscar-winning movie star to the average Joe on the street, and were silenced or ostracized.

The sites led me to more sites where I read about the genocide in Darfur, the lawlessness and civil war in Somalia, the AIDS epidemic wiping out a whole generation of Africans. Hurricane Katrina, Britain flooding, extreme weather conditions affecting extreme poverty in the Third World, and the famine in Ethiopia, which had worsened since the first Live Aid in 1988.

I slammed the laptop lid down; I couldn't take anymore. Was this for real? The planet's situation had got so much worse, not better as I had imagined it would, and I felt so helpless. One positive thing was that there hadn't been a nuclear war but from what I had read, it seemed like the world was only moments away from it happening. *Those CND marches didn't work then*, I thought.

I wiped my tears, and picked up a broadsheet paper, the

front of which spoke about new regulations on cloning human DNA. I took a deep breath and opened it up to the middle section. It read 'Hunger. Strikes. Riots. The food crisis bites' in big black bold type surrounded by images of people from all over the world scrambling for handouts from aid aeroplanes and queuing up outside stores to buy their food in bulk, not knowing when the next delivery would be.

Photographs of long queues of cars waiting to fill their tanks at petrol stations sat next to pictures of empty supermarket shelves. I gulped down the strong wave of fear that threatened to engulf me and fought back the tears. It was futile. I couldn't take anymore. I threw down the paper, pulled the duvet cover over my head, and let out one long scream. I lay there for what felt like an eternity and screamed and screamed and screamed until my voice went hoarse.

What could I possibly do, me, one of six and a half billion people? How was I going to save the world? I lay on the bed and sobbed, cried for the planet and all its apparently unsolvable problems. I had woken up in a *Blade Runner, Soylent Green, Logan's Run*, Orwellian nightmare and I was petrified. I wanted to go home.

If Adult Naomi knew this about the world, why did she selfishly bring a child into it? I felt resentment release into the bitter water that flowed from my eyes. I suddenly hated Adult Naomi for becoming a victim of greed, excess, and consumption. Was this what had caused her crap life and her reason for leaving the building, leaving me to pick up the pieces of this dismal smegging life she'd created? Well, I resolved then and there, I wasn't going to end up like her; I was going to figure this stuff out and do everything in my power to make things better before I left.

I squeezed my eyes shut and tried to force my brain to forget, to forget everything it had read or seen. It didn't happen; instead I saw a scene from *Back to the Future* where Doc Brown was telling Marty not to leave the house in 1959, as it could have serious consequences on the future. I opened my eyes. Had I done something wrong in 1992? Had I made a decision back then that had dire consequences for my future and now I was being made to live out the nightmare of an alien world filled with strange technology and smegged-up ideas?

I felt like one of those tattered notes in a bottle drifting on an endless wave, lost. Would I ever leave the year 2008, and what would happen to me if I couldn't? The many questions swirling around my mind eventually collapsed into a faint din humming in the empty space that once housed Adult Naomi's memories.

Exhausted, I lay back and closed my aching eyes.

I woke up hours later. Still in the future and still fifteen. I felt well sad. The room was dark. I lay in the large bed, staring at the grey walls. Images of the world played in reverse in my mind, from the last newspaper article to the two aeroplanes speeding into tall glass buildings. Fear began to stir in the pit of my belly, but the shrill tone of the mobile phone jump-started my heart into an adrenaline-fuelled alertness. The flashing screen told me it was Simone.

'Hiya, babe. How you feeling? How's your head?' She

sounded relaxed, calm. Her voice instantly soothed my panic.

'I'm okay,' I said, still a bit freaked out.

'You don't sound it, *chica*.'

'Did you know the planet is running out of food?' I started to cry again; where the tears were coming from, I had no frickin' idea.

'What?'

'Yeah, I read it in the newspaper and all this other stuff, like Mum was right about Nostradamus. Sim, the world is ending,' I sobbed.

'What? Oh, Nay, seriously, don't believe everything you read in the papers; you already know it's just a lot of fear mongering.'

'I do?' I was confused.

'Yeah, you are, like, one of those people who doesn't read or watch the news. You say half of it is magnified half-truths and that no one ever reports the good things humans do, and you think there's a bigger conspiracy going on to keep everyone scared and ignorant. You believe it's all one big set-up.'

'Are you squerious?' I asked her. First the vegan stuff, now a conspiracy theorist. Adult Naomi was a hippie after all.

'Yeah, babe. Nay, put down the papers and step away from the propaganda. Don't believe the hype. Remember?'

Those four words, *don't believe the hype*, reminded me of a Public Enemy rap song that condemned such sensationalism and fear mongering and told my generation to think for ourselves.

'I need to smell me some teen spirit.' I smiled and started to laugh.

'Exactly,' Simone agreed.

'Thanks, sis,' I said, grateful she had called.

'Listen, we've been out all day and are completely soaked. Leo wants to stay the night. Is that okay?'

It was a relief to hear. I didn't want him to see me this way but guessed I wouldn't be able to hide my real feelings from him. I wanted the space to clear my head and straighten my thoughts.

'Oh, okay, sorted. Sim, you are totally safe.'

'No problem, and I'll cook tomorrow and bring your dinner up when I bring him home.'

'Wicked.'

'And Nay?'

'Yeah?'

'Chill the hell out and stop with the worrying. Nothing is ever as bad as it seems,' she said.

'Okay.' I wanted to believe her, but my apocalyptic cynicism told me otherwise.

'Go and eat some cottage cheese and watch a movie.'

What a good idea. I hadn't eaten anything since that morning and needed some respite from the mental assault my brain had just experienced.

I hung the phone up and, still wrapped in my duvet, I went downstairs to the kitchen. There I buttered two slices of brown bread, heaped a large dollop of cottage cheese on one and poured myself a glass of orange juice. I sat down on the sofa, switched on the TV, avoiding the news and the weird reality shows until I found UKTV Gold. It was a marathon of old episodes of a comedy called *Absolutely Fabulous*. I had never seen it before but as a huge French and Saunders fan I was intrigued. And as I watched these two shallow, self-absorbed, fashion-obsessed women and their cigarette-smoking, drunken adventures in PR, trying to avoid an exasperated straight-laced daughter, I avoided Adult Naomi's life in much the same way, dodging the questions I didn't want the answers to. My dark mood lifted. I settled in for the night and as I watched and laughed at the funny one-liners, I began to chill and, for a short while, forgot what being *global* felt like.

6

The Secret Diary of Naomi Jacobs

The motion of the ocean
is just like emotion:
you've got to
let it flow,
and put that in your journal.

C. B.

I sat in the cold room and stared at the walls while the doctor tapped the keys of the computer. It felt well weird. In his dark blue suit and matching tie he reminded me of Mr Jervis, my maths teacher, a cross between Albert Einstein and Homer Simpson. I couldn't stand Jumpin' Jack Jervis and his dragon breath, his foul temper, his wild hair and his skin with this, like, strange yellow tint. And this doctor wasn't much better.

'And how long have you experienced this, er, "memory loss"?' The doctor peered at me over his silver-rimmed glasses. I knew from the tone of his voice he hadn't believed a word I'd said.

'Since Thursday.'

'And you don't remember a thing?'

I shook my head, then nodded. 'No . . . I mean, yes . . . I mean, no . . . I don't remember some stuff and I do remember other stuff.' I was beginning to wish I'd brought my sister in.

'Well, what *do* you remember?' he asked.

'Erm, numbers, like phone numbers, and I know my bank number and I think I remember how to drive; I kind of remember my son. Well, I feel I do.'

'You *feel* you do?' He sighed heavily.

I nodded. The words coming out of my mouth sounded cracked so I pulled out the paper and read the words I had written the night before. 'I think I've lost my episodic memory.' I took a deep breath. 'But my semantic memory is okay.'

'I beg your pardon?' It was as if I had just spoken in an obscure language from a remote village in the Himalayas. The language I *was* speaking was called 'neurological psychology' and I was a long way from home.

'I think I might have something called transient global amnesia.'

He tried to disguise a laugh underneath a loud cough. 'Transient global amnesia,' he repeated. 'And what makes you think that?'

I explained as best I could, starting with waking up in the future and ending with me furiously researching amnesia. Given the traumatic events, I hadn't been able to wait any longer. I had woken yet again from more bad dreams, sweating in a pool of my own frickin' despair. Frustrated by my fear of a world I didn't understand and worried about brain damage, I'd decided to take things into my own hands and try and figure out myself what was wrong with me. Maybe deep down I had felt that I would be laughed out of the doctor's surgery unless I could come up with an explanation as to why I was fifteen again.

At first my research on amnesia had ended in futility as most of the explanations for memory loss centred around car accidents and lobotomies, neither of which I'd had. The words 'permanent brain damage' had imprinted on my mind and then rung in my ears as I'd slammed the laptop lid down in frustration. But as I paced the house, racking my possibly damaged brain, it had come to me that if it wasn't physical, then it could be mental or, more to the point, psychological.

And here was where Adult Naomi came to the rescue. It was the first time I was actually grateful for the decision she had made to study psychology. Looking at her university books, it seemed that she had every book available on the brain and how it affected behaviour. It was tough-going – there was all this stuff on neurological and psychological theory that I so didn't get. Everything from how people choose their partners to why some people get addicted to drugs and others don't. Still, as much as I didn't get it, I needed to know. So I had taken all of Sunday while Leo was still with Simone and half the night when he was sleeping and Simone had gone to bed to go through the mountain of books Adult Naomi had left behind. I had almost given in until I came across a small textbook, which included a chapter called 'Loss of episodic memory in retrograde amnesia'. It described something called 'psychogenic amnesia', where there was commonly a past history of 'transient organic memory loss'. I'd had to look in a dictionary to understand the words, but when I did, it had made me wonder whether this had happened to Adult Naomi before. It also stated that this psychogenic amnesia could be situation-specific – brought on by a car accident or sexual abuse in childhood – and in those cases, there are brief gaps in memory for the episode. Alternatively, it said that psychogenic amnesia could be 'global', encompassing the whole of a person's past, and could occur in so-called 'fugue' episodes.

The author outlined the three known case studies where transient global amnesia had lasted longer than twenty-four to forty-eight hours. I was fascinated. The story that stood out for me was that of a teenager, a nineteen-year-old male university student, who was found in a city park a few days before his exams were due to start. In addition to the stress of his exams, he had also lost his grandmother who he had been quite close to. Doctors took witness accounts from those who had been with him from the start. He had lost his autobiographical memory and his memory of public events. His recovery of memory function was monitored and it took four weeks for the retrograde amnesia to end.

The two other known cases both involved men; one had transient global amnesia for eight months, the other for a few days. What I noticed was that they had all suffered some form of heavy loss in their lives and were experiencing long and intense periods of something called 'stress' before they lost their memories.

The relief I experienced when I finished reading these stories was how I imagined it felt to be released by a large boa constrictor before it crushed the living daylights out of you – well grateful. I still didn't understand how I could remember my bank card number or Katie's phone number but further on in the chapter I came across something called 'semantic memory' – where all of a person's automatic memories are stored, having been formed through repetitive use, such as memories of phone numbers, how to drive or of using the same bus route every morning – and 'episodic memory', which was connected to all the major experiences in your life such as births, deaths, marriages or significant relationships, as well as the life-changing events that people have, which affect them on a more profound level.

It was difficult to take it all in but I eventually understood that these different types of memory were both hidden in the subconscious, and used if and when needed. Of course memories fade as we get older and details are lost, but we are reminded of the special events in our lives through sound (a wedding song), touch (a child's hug), smell (Mum's roast potatoes), sight (a faded Polaroid), or taste (Granddad's eggnog). What we remember, what our brains choose to retain, is simply what makes each person unique. The author explained that we can all have different memories of the same events because our perspectives will always be different. Whether it's through one of our five senses, our dreams, or even a deeper intuition, human beings remember what we need to survive and we discard what we don't.

My brain had no emotional memories of the last seventeen years. By the time I had finished reading this book, I knew this as fact. Now, here in this surgery, all I needed to do was convince the doctor and get it checked out.

The doctor had been listening patiently. 'So, let me get this straight,' he said. 'You can't remember anything from the last seventeen years, but you remembered how to get here and how to get money at the cashpoint?'

'Well, my sister brought me,' I replied.

'I see.' He turned back to his computer and continued to tap the keys.

I bit my lip. This appointment wasn't going the way I had expected it to. 'I . . . I know what it sounds like, but I really think I have amnesia,' I stammered, tears starting to form.

'Oh, you do, do you?' His bearded face couldn't hide his smirk.

'Yes, I think I've been very stressed and then I woke up and I'm fifteen. I can't remember how I got here.'

'But you said your sister brought you.'

I looked at him, wondering why he was being such a total tosspot. I was about to start ramping*.

'No, I mean here, Manchester, this life . . .' I said. 'I don't think I have a brain tumour, or brain damage, because I haven't, like, you know, had an accident or anything, but do you think I should maybe see a specialist? Like, in a hospital?'

This time he laughed. 'A brain tumour? I don't think so. In fact, Ms Jacobs, I think this is all in your imagination and I think you need to go home, have a nice cup of tea, and get some rest.'

Was this guy serious? I stared at him. According to this smeg for brains of a doctor sitting in front of me, waking up and still being fifteen years old, when I clearly wasn't, was all in my imagination and all's I needed to fix it was a cup of tea? I sat and stared at him until the tears filled my eyes and distorted his yellow face. He stared back defiantly.

---

* *Ramping/ramp* – to act up or start shit, regardless of the consequences.

I blinked away the tears. 'But I can't remember the last seventeen years. I . . . I don't know how I got here.'

'Well, you said you woke up here the other morning.'

'Yeah.' I was giving face now, full of serious attitude; I so needed to chip.

'So you have been here all along.'

'Yes, I know THAT! But I don't remember *being* here. This is what I'm trying to say to you!'

'Yes, well, like I said before . . .' He sighed and rubbed his large Tefal scientist Homer Simpson fod*. 'You just need to go home and rest and I'm sure things will go back to normal soon. Do you need more sleeping tablets?'

'What?' My face started to burn.

'I see by your notes you take sleeping tablets.'

I wanted to dive out of my chair across the desk, grab his big slaphead and shake it into the reality of the living hell I was experiencing.

'I don't, no, I don't.'

'Well, it says here, your last prescription was for sleeping tablets.' He pressed a button on his computer keypad and the grey printer next to his desk began to whir.

'You need a good night's sleep and some rest.'

The printer spewed out a green prescription, which he quickly signed and handed to me. I stared at him for a moment longer, not knowing what to do. He stuck out the paper further, indicating for me to take it from his hands.

I grabbed the prescription from him and stood up. I wiped my face. 'This is so stale,' I mumbled.

---

* *Fod* – forehead.

'You're welcome.' He gave me a fake smile.

I stormed out of the room into the waiting room and marched up to the receptionist's desk. Simone stood up, her smile quickly fading when she noticed the pissed-off look on my face.

'Can I help you?' the blonde-haired woman asked me from behind the glass partition.

'Yes, I was wondering if you could tell me which doctor I usually see?'

She sighed, shook her head and turned to her computer.

'What's your name?'

I told her. She read the screen for a few seconds and then turned to me.

'You normally see Doctor Rahman, but he's away on annual leave.'

'When will he be back?' I asked her.

Simone put her hand on my back and rubbed it softly.

'Two weeks' time,' she replied. Anticipating my next question, she added, 'But you can't make an appointment to see him until he's here.'

'Fine, thank you.' I turned from the desk and walked straight out of the building.

Simone followed me into the car park. 'Are you okay, babe?'

I shook my head. As soon as the cool air hit me, a large barrel of shame churned inside my stomach, mixing it with fear and producing anger.

'He said I was imagining it and all's I needed was a good night's sleep.'

'What the . . .' She quickened her step and caught up with me. 'What shall we do, babe?' She looked scared.

I burst into tears. 'I don't want to go to hospital, Sim.'

She put her arm around my shoulder and walked me to the car. 'I know, *chica*, I know. We can go back in and demand an answer.'

'No, he's not my doctor. He's a smeghead, a pecker neck. What does he know?'

We stood outside the car and I took a big gulp of air. 'Has this happened to me before, Sim?' I sobbed.

'What? No, I don't think so, but, Nay, you have been through some serious stuff at times, stuff that's really stressed you out.'

I wiped my eyes and opened the car door. 'Well, whether that knobhead believes me or not, I know what to do.'

'What?'

'Stop stressing for a start and I just need some time. Two weeks, until my doctor gets back. Let me see him first and if nothing's changed, I'll ask him to send me straight to hospital, straight to a brain doctor.'

'Okay, babe. Well, whatever you need, Nay, I'm here for you, okay?' She smiled and gave me a hug. 'We'll get through this.'

I hiccupped a last sob into her arms and swallowed down the fear.

I had been hoping the appointment would have solved this amnesia problem and somehow helped the memories come back, as they eventually did for the student with transient global anaemia. But it didn't. If anything, it made things ten times worse. Maybe the doctor was right. Maybe it was in my imagination. Maybe I would just fall asleep and wake up back in 1992 like I originally thought. Maybe I was just going crazy – the thirty-two-year-old me had lost her mind and my fifteen-year-old self had replaced her. Or maybe I had a mental illness. Maybe I was schizophrenic. I felt sick. Whatever was happening, I didn't want anyone in Adult Naomi's life to know, least of all my parents. So far I'd managed not to involve them, but if I went to hospital they would have to be told.

Simone was there for me. I knew that she would totally do anything I asked. But I felt really alone and under pressure to sort things out. I knew the problem wasn't in my imagination, but I figured if it was in my brain then it was in my mind, and although I couldn't do anything about my brain, I could do something about my mind.

On the way back to that small house on that tree-lined street, I knew it was time. Time for me – fifteen-year-old Nay – to truly find a way into Adult Naomi's house. The house I had seen that night in my mind, just before I fell asleep. The house I thought about every time I searched for a memory. Maybe I would be able to find her and she would be able to help me. I knew that the memories were hidden somewhere inside of me and, if I was brave enough, I might somehow find them and make things better. I could fix what was broken and change everything. This, I hoped, would be the fuel needed to propel my time-travelling arse back to the year 1992 and create the space needed for Adult Naomi to come back.

I wrestled all night with my conscience. The responsibility I felt for finding Adult Naomi grew with each passing hour. Every time I closed my eyes, I couldn't help but turn to the house and stare as hard as I could at it. I felt like I needed to get in now, but I knew the door was locked and I was scared. What if I couldn't get in ever? What if I did and she wasn't there? The urgent need for me to gain access would increase but then I'd find myself fighting my insistence to know, telling myself it wasn't my business and that everything would go back to normal soon.

But where was I to go? I couldn't remember anything and I knew I wouldn't be able to survive on automatic memory alone. Nobody was gonna help me. There was no magic pill or potion I could take to make me shrink small enough to climb through a window and gain access to the house.

But there had to be a way in.

Eventually, I turned over and as I was falling asleep, I decided to give up and go to the hospital the next day.

That night I dreamt of butterflies – well, one butterfly in particular. I couldn't tell what kind of butterfly it was but it felt familiar. It lay in front of me while I was walking with someone, a faceless person, but someone I had a feeling I knew. We were on a deserted beach. The butterfly was injured; there were small pools of water and drops of blood surrounding it, and I kept thinking, *If I don't help it, it will drown.* I couldn't see or tell where it was hurt. I just knew I had to get it home and clean it, so I picked it up and put it into my pocket. The person with me told me not to put it there in case it couldn't breathe, but I knew it would be safe with me. And then a massive wave rushed up from the sea and washed over everything, taking us with it.

Sack it, I thought as I woke up the next morning. *I know the problem and I'm gonna apply the solution; I'm not some dumb kid. I mean, when I was nine, my teacher told my mum I was three years above my reading age and whenever anything needs figuring out in our house everyone always says 'Our Nay will do it', so yeah, I'm gonna figure it out.*

With this weird feeling that it was somehow my responsibility to help Adult Naomi, I decided I was going to get the memories back, and would begin by reading all of the journals she had left behind, twenty years' of diaries to be exact. Simone was going to stay with me until she was convinced I could cope with Leo and the day-to-day running of the house. I knew it wouldn't be hard; the house was small and clean and I had babysat for kids since the age of twelve, so I was used to it, and Leo felt like the little brother I had never had.

Although I was eager to meet the brother I did have, JJ, we decided Simone would take over communication with the outside world for me, while I took the time to find Adult Naomi. How hard could it be? I didn't have a job, I didn't wanna drive, even though I could remember how to. The exams were weeks away, and by that time she would be back and able to deal with them. In the meantime, until I could get to see her real doctor or wake up back in 1992, I would forget the future world and instead delve into Adult Naomi's world, with the help of her diaries.

My sister had gone to work and Leo was at school. Apart from the odd car driving past, the street had grown quiet, leaving me in solitude. I was kinda nervous, but intrigued. I wanted to know, what could have possibly happened to her, to me, to us?

I began with the last one written the night before I had woken up in the future, to see what it could tell me.

I took a deep breath.

1.37 a.m. 17 April 2008

I jogged today, only to the corner shop, but I jogged and it was nice. It's different jogging in the street rather than at the gym. You feel like you're getting somewhere. I might try the park tomorrow. I want to start running again; figure I can't run from here, I can't run from the past, but jogging is as good as it gets, plus it'll help me quit smoking, keep me fit and keep my mind clear for my exams. Maybe I'll run myself to sleep ☺. It's been an emotional day. I'm exhausted.

Maybe I'm not ready to let go just yet. I know I need to and I will – I want to – but I feel these exams, writing all of these exams, is part of the process. Part of the process of finally letting go of the past, writing about the past, living in the past. And maybe I can start to live in the present, looking to the future. I need a new beginning. Yes, maybe my new beginning will be creating a life without the past getting involved! The power of yesterday, hey? Except I know, as Tolle says, the power of Now is even more powerful. I just wish I understood that. Still, I'm glad I honoured how I felt today and was honest with Katie. I needed to just let go and cry it all out, you know?

I kind of freaked out when I realized I hadn't done anything for anybody for a whole week (apart from Leo). It felt really selfish. I didn't want to say anything because I was afraid of looking bad, afraid of what Caroline would think of me. Why? Isn't it about time? She, with her belief in self-empowerment, would approve. She was the one who told me in front of the class that I had to learn how

*to say NO! Isn't this a new beginning for me? A fresh
start. I will cleanse my body of the past, I will . . .*

What the smeg? What the frick was self-empowerment?
And why did she need to take a class? And why couldn't she
tell people no? I couldn't believe she was afraid of what other
people thought of her. At least she was exercising and had
vowed to quit smoking – as long as I had control of Adult
Naomi's body she wouldn't start again.

I read the remainder of the entry and questioned every
word written.

*I know Henri is part of me letting go. Okay, so I did, I
did visualize us being in each other's future and I've never
done that before, but at least I know I can do it now. I
can be with a man and plan a future. I keep thinking of
the dream I had about that gorgeous tall man I met on
holiday. It wasn't Henri, though, which I'm a bit gutted
about. But maybe Henri was my preparation, my stepping
stone. And as the saying goes,* All my mistakes are
stepping stones to my success. *I mean, I know I was
meant to meet him, and now I know I needed to be
rescued by a man who looked and smoked like my dad,
which is so Freudian. I finally got what I had wanted
since I was a child. Got what I had been waiting for. I got
what I wanted, the man to come and rescue me and kiss
the boo boo, make the pain go away, and you know what,
he did and the boo boo was still there. I think I am the
only one that can make it feel better and kiss it. Me,
myself and I! I think! Can I? Anyway, I listened to my*

inner child and took her advice, watched P.S. I Love You
*– ha-ha-ha funny (although Gerald Butler's Irish accent
is awful and you just can't do that to one of the sexiest
accents on the planet). I laughed, I cried, ultimately . . .
I kissed my boo boo . . .*

Okay, stop. What the bloody hell was the boo boo? And
who was this inner child? I put the diary down and it sat open
on the bed, silent. No answer to my questions other than,
If you wanna know, Nay, read some more. So I took a deep
breath, picked the book up, and stared at the black writing
scrawled across the pages. I told myself I could handle it. It
wasn't my life and I could deal.

I was *sooooo* not prepared for what came next.

*I'm aware that the dream is me doing my best to repel
Henri (Dad 1) and am looking for a secure attachment to
future possible boyfriend (Dad 2). Unless I have come full
circle again in the realization that I can and will meet my
two dads in one man!*

Okay, I thought. *So, firstly, what's with the American sitcom
crap about My Two Dads? And secondly, why the smeg would I
want to end up with a man like my dads? I mean, they are cool
and everything, but I kinda know that I am not gonna be with
a man like either of them for various reasons FULL STOP!*
When I read my future husband checklist . . .
Oh Jeez!

*. . . I embody most of those qualities, things like sensitive
and caring, a good listener, and I've been told I'm strong,*

*and I know if he ticks all the boxes or comes close to
embodying most if not all of those qualities, then he's the
one for me.*

But why?

*Let me peruse them for a moment . . . Henri got nineteen
out of thirty. I gave him 'has lovely hair' because judging
by his old pictures, he did have lovely hair and I did like
touching his bald head a lot.*

Oh dear God. I breathed in hard. *I think I'm gonna hurl!*

*He has ten of Dad 1 and nine of Dad 2. Well, I suppose
what is true is that one stuck around and one ran away.*

What? Wait! What? My stepdad ran away?

I put the diary down and picked up the phone. Simone
answered after the second ring. 'What's up, sis? Everything
okay?'

'Yeah, I just . . . Sim, did Joe run away?' I had assumed Joe
(Joseph), my stepfather, was still around somewhere, maybe
even in London, where apparently Evelyn (my mum) lived.

'Nay, I can't really talk right now. I'm at work.' She sounded
tense.

'I know . . . you don't have to tell me what happened. Just
answer yes or no.'

'Yes.'

'Wow! So, like, he's still in our life, right? Does he visit or
do we go and see him?'

'Nay, seriously, we can talk about this when I come up after work.'

Why was she being so cryptic? It was a simple question that required a simple yes or no answer. 'Sim, just quickly tell me.'

She whispered into the phone. 'You haven't seen him since you were eighteen. He disappeared nearly fifteen years ago and no one has seen him since. Some people think he's dead; others say he faked his own death, stole millions, and changed his identity. Maybe it wasn't just weed he was selling, and in the end he got caught up in the serious drug world and it killed him? Who knows, sis? Bottom line is, he left.'

I laughed. Simone didn't.

'I've got to go; we'll talk about it when I come up.' And with that, she hung up her phone and left me standing staring at the floor, mouth gaping like a fish out of water. The words *you haven't seen him since you were eighteen* echoed in my ears. I shook them out of my head and came up for air. They were immediately replaced with *disappeared nearly fifteen years ago. Why?* And my mind screamed, *where the bloody hell is he?*

I sat back down on the bed in shock and stared at the different journals scattered across the floor. They would tell me and, if I read on, I knew I would eventually find the answers to all of my questions. So I placed the phone on the table next to the bed, picked up the journal, and lay down.

I think I've just figured out why my inner child was so attached to Henri. Have I really got to make a choice and stick to it? Joseph or Art? If I was a little girl and I had to choose, I would've run to my dad, no question. If I was a

*teenager and had a choice I would have run to Joseph
and I did . . .*

I did?

*. . . Yes, okay, it was for money! But I still turned to him.
In the end, though, when I was a teenager I ran back to
my dad; if I hadn't, I wouldn't have survived everything
that happened and I wouldn't be here today and, well,
when I was in the hostel . . .*

I was in a hostel?

*I ran to my dad again and that Christmas with him and
JJ and Leo was lovely, even though I wasn't talking to
Simone; it was greatly needed! But then why did I dream
about that tall guy if I am so in love with Henri and why
did I start taking coke again?*

Hold up, wait a minute, rewind, come again? I did what?
Did I read right? Did she write right? She started taking
coke again? As in cocaine? As in blow? As in powder? As in
that crap Danniella Westbrook from *EastEnders* shoved up
her nose until it caved in?! I was horrified, mortified, disappointed, and dumbfounded all in one big ball of disbelief.

*Yes, maybe because I realized that my dad couldn't give
me what I needed emotionally. No, maybe I realized or
felt I couldn't get through university homeless anyway!
But in essence, being there did give me something I
needed because I got through my dissertation, cocaine*

*and all! So back to the original question, do I really have
to make a choice about which one was the better dad
and hope he embodies most of the qualities of that dad
or, like the relationship book says, the qualities of the one
who stuck around, the one who was reliable, the one who
was dependable? Which of course has been Art. Well,
whatever the answer, there was creativity in both of them,
whether it was music or painting; there is no creativity in
Henri – I mean, of course there is; there is in everybody,
he just hasn't found it yet – and that is the most
important quality to possess. I mean, that he must own.
Creativity! Yes. Am I creative, though? Oh, who knows!*

I put the diary down. My mind was reeling and I felt sick
– trying to digest the words was seriously making me want to
hurl my breakfast. Something had to come out, but instead I
choked down the sour taste in my mouth and said the words
out loud. 'She was homeless while she was at university and she
did cocaine while she wrote her dissertation and she broke up
with her boyfriend and was obsessed with her relationships
with my dads and . . .' I stopped. I felt really embarrassed. This
wasn't my life; this couldn't be the woman I had turned into.

I paced the floor, wracking my brain, searching for any
memory. Something that could explain what I had just read.
But all I could think was, *Who the hell is Adult Naomi?*

Like partygoers being refused entry by a bouncer at a
nightclub door, my questions were turned away answerless.
My head started to hurt but I had to keep going. I decided to
use the last diary entry as a starting point and work my way
backwards.

I opened the diary randomly and read an entry.

2 October 2007

It is 3.20 a.m. and I've curled up with a spliff and my insomnia! My nose is blocked, presumably from the crap coke I had at the weekend. Bloody Ajax giving me the Columbian flu. Slightly bemused with myself for having taken it in the first place, and yet not at the same time, because you know what? I tried to write in here while under the influence and it all came out weird, my handwriting and everything! Seeing that made it clear what the cocaine is doing to my brain. Anyway, I am listening to the tunes that will hopefully transport my mind to another place and take me out of this life right now and drop me somewhere in the near future.

I'm reading a book, a misery memoir, still figuring out why I even bought it in the first place as all it has achieved is making me more miserable. Why do they tell you everything that happened to them and tell you that they got over it but never tell you how exactly? Never really get to the inside of the person's mind and how they dealt with all of the crap, how they healed it? You don't just wake up one day and everything is okay – life doesn't work like that. Still, maybe reading it has given me the push I needed to deal with the painful energy that has manifested as my inner child and help me try to heal everything into wholeness. Will I ever?

It hangs around like a bad smell – the manipulation and intimidation that has played a big part in my life – and every day I struggle to complete the day feeling

*whole, loved and right within myself. Will a day ever
come when I will? And well, frankly, since moving into
this house it seems to have become harder; the transition
to settling down again in this city has been far from easy,
coupled with the sudden loss of two cousins, the second so
far removed from my life that I was searching for the
news report about Sean being murdered before to see if it
would sink in that he was dead. Killed, gone, murdered,
and how amazing it all is. Is amazing the right word?
Maybe bewildering is it! No, shocking! Yes, shocking.*

*Evelyn is visiting Simone this weekend and I have
come to the conclusion that I am not running away by
going to Bradford with Rhonda to see her cousins. I am
protecting my inner child from harm. I am recognizing
my vulnerability, because I have no job, I am not settled
into my home or way of life, not right within myself,
certainly not strong or brave enough to deal with her.
And you know what? That's okay. It's okay to admit that
sometimes you just ain't got the balls to do it, as much as
you may want to. For fuck's sake, I'm not superwoman,
and as much as I would like to see Simone, I have no
energy to smile up in their faces and play like everything
in my life is okay. I'd most probably go postal. It would all
end up being really dramatic and . . . oh, I don't even
want to think about it, but right now, my not being there
is saying what I need to say, which is, I ain't ready for you
yet. I'm still reeling from the last whirlwind you caused
when you were like the Tasmanian Devil, leaving me with
a bitch of a headache and my life in tatters. No, I need
more time. This is Evelyn's and Simone's thing, not mine.*

Charlie dying was out of my control. It was natural causes. I had a choice to be at the funeral and deal with The Sisters; I chose that. I have a choice to be here when Eve's here; I choose not to be.

I couldn't believe it. Even though his dad and mine hadn't spoken in years, in spite of being brothers, I did meet Sean once when he was little; but murdered – gosh, his poor mum. And my cousin Charlie had died. I had grown up with Charlie, because his mum was Eve's sister. Had he died because of his epilepsy?

My heart thumped in my chest with an uneven beat; I swallowed, closed the diary, and began to cry.

I couldn't read anymore. I didn't understand half of the things Adult Naomi had written and I needed to talk to someone about it before I sent myself mental with questions. In the meantime, I had to wait for Simone to return from work and get myself together as Leo was on his way home from school. I needed to pretend everything was okay.

Moments later, Leo came through the door as happy as any ten-year-old could be. He swung his bag down and went straight to the fridge, where he grabbed a juice carton. I stood in the kitchen, watching the way he moved. His mannerisms and facial expressions majorly wigged me out, but in, like, a really good way.

'You okay, Mum?' He looked apprehensive.

'What? Yeah, I'm cool, cool as a cucumber.' I smiled and put my thumbs up and reached in for a drink also. I couldn't let him think something was up.

'Err, okay.' He laughed.

I laughed with him, remembering what sounded totally normal to me must have seemed totally wack to him. I was, after all, a thirty-two-year-old mother, even though I felt like a fifteen-year-old babysitting big sister. I think he knew something wasn't fine. His answer was to suggest we play a game.

'Do you wanna go on the Wii?'

I spat out my juice all over the kitchen floor. Leo found this hilarious.

'Your what? What the smegnacious is a Wee?'

'Smegnacious!' He giggled. 'The Nintendo Wii, Mum.' At this, he left the kitchen and ran upstairs.

I grabbed the cloth and wiped up the apple juice from the floor. I knew what a Nintendo was – a small grey box with two joy pads connected to it; you were no one until you'd taken on the Super Mario brothers in boiler suits and kicked Donkey Kong's arse. But what was the Wee bit?

Leo returned with a bright white box that looked nothing like a Nintendo. It had no buttons and, it seemed, no letterbox-type slot to stick your game in. I watched as he connected it to the back of the television. He arranged the box on the floor and pressed a button on a white, funny-shaped remote. A drawer slid open; he placed a disc inside, and it swallowed it. The words *Wii Sport* appeared on the mega TV screenage and he handed me a remote.

'What do you wanna play first?' He smiled at me.

'Err.' I was stumped. I didn't even know how to work the object he had given me.

'We'll play tennis.' He made a few gestures and pressed his

thumb on the remote and these funny-looking little people appeared on the screen.

'Choose your avatar, Mum.'

'You do it, I like yours better.' I shoved the remote into his free hand.

'Okay.' Seeming to accept this reasoning, he took the remote from me and I watched, eyes glued to the mega screen-age, as he chose hair, skin colour, and the clothing that best represented me. He then named it Nay. I had to pretend like I knew what he was doing, but I really wanted to scream, *Oh my dayz! What the hell is this futuristic box thing where the players look like you and it's got no buttons?* What he showed me next almost floored me. To imagine in the future you would actually stand in front of a television, use a remote control as a tennis racket and play an opponent as if you were on a court; it was something I expected to see in a frickin' George Lucas film, not in the living room of my house. And certainly not in my lifetime.

I followed Leo's example and every time he swung his arm with the remote in his hand, the ball would bat to the other side. My side. I missed the serve several times while screaming and squealing like a total spazoid. I couldn't get my head around the crazy reality of me interacting with the television. I expected Arnold Schwarzenegger to appear in a latex tennis suit and pull off his fake head while running through a maze screaming, *It's the future, Nay, and your son has just initiated you . . . Oh, and I'll be back.*

We played for most of the afternoon. He changed games from tennis to bowling to golf and then boxing. I laughed so hard I almost wet myself (apparently this had something to do with having a 9lb baby, Katie told me one night). Leo was a veteran at the games, so I lost most of the time, but my competitive streak came out and I refused to give up. It was the first time since I had woken up in the future that I was actually having fun. When we took a break and flopped down on the sofa, I looked over at a sweating, giggling Leo.

Adult Naomi had done one right thing with her life. He was very smart and fun to be around and I could see why everyone was so proud of him. The words 'I love you' burst out of me and I gave him an awkward hug and a kiss on the cheek. His response was to push me off him and wipe his cheek in disgust while still giggling. He jumped up off the sofa, said, 'Better take my uniform off,' and disappeared out of the door.

Oh Jeez, yeah, I forgot. Mums tell kids to take their uniforms off when they get home from school, don't they?

Leo popped his head back around the door and said, 'I love you too, Mum,' and ran back up the stairs.

Nice one! Top one! Sawwwted! As I sat basking in the glow of this new slush puppy squidgy feeling, my mind turned to Eve, my own mother. A woman I had nicknamed the Wicked Witch of the West Midlands and assured everyone who would listen that although I loved her (being her daughter, there wasn't much choice in the matter), if I wasn't born to her, we would not be friends and I would never have anyone in my life remotely like her.

Why weren't we ever like this? I thought. *Wasn't I a cool kid like Leo?*

I just never got my mum. I never understood her love and was scared because I couldn't figure her out. I had a sense that there was a time when she had loved me, but all of that had changed when we left Art and the life we knew in Liverpool and moved to Wolverhampton when I was five years old. As I got older our relationship grew more intense, aggressive, and became filled with so many insane arguments that I was convinced she hated me and wished I had never been born. I often lay awake at night wondering if she'd prefer it if I was dead.

And then it hit me. Why was Eve so far away from Adult Naomi? Why wasn't she a part of her grandchild's life? Mine and Simone's lives? What had happened?

I followed Leo upstairs and sat in the bedroom, reading another diary entry while he was getting changed. I *sooooo* wished I hadn't, because he reappeared moments later and I had to swallow down the sadness I was feeling.

20 October 2006

My first night in this awful place, and there is only one question I have. Am I being punished? Did I do something so terribly wrong that I deserve the life I am living? Do you want me to suffer? I don't think I can do this anymore. I do my best and yet it's never good enough? Over and over, I make the same mistakes and choose that which is so, so, so wrong for me. I have failed Leo; I have failed at life; I am a failure. I must have done some bad things to be punished in this way. My karma must be so negative, so full of pain. I must have hurt so many people because I am hurting enough for a hundred souls.

The past couple of years, in fact, my whole life has been full of unreliable, untrustworthy people, family and

friends whom I have loved unconditionally; I have tried
to express this to them and yet I am constantly being
attacked, shamed or ridiculed for being me. I just don't
get it! Why? Why did I come back here? To this madness,
this insanity, to a city so grey and depressing? To live in
a hostel with my nine-year-old and beg pennies off the
social? My home, Greece, my business and my car are all
gone. I miss my home so much. I miss the safety and
security of my living room, and my sofa, my bed. I miss
my home.

All the choices, all the mistakes that I have made, and
I end up here, in this place. We'll most probably be sent
to a crap flat on some fucked-up council estate; there'll
be me on my own trying to keep Leo safe, and my control-
freak sister (I am so bloody angry with her) who thinks
I'm always in crisis and needs me to make a plan! When I
think things can get no worse, that I can sink no lower,
they do and I do. I'm being punished, right? This is a cruel
joke; this is a nightmare and I haven't woken up yet. So if
I'm being punished, make it stop, please make it stop.
Please take me tonight, please. I can't wake up tomorrow.
I can't go through another day. I don't have the strength
anymore. I can't do this anymore, I just can't, I really
can't.

Sadness wedged in the back of my throat like a piece of dry
bread and remained stuck there until Simone walked into the
house. I was happy to see her and she was happy to see me.
She made us spaghetti bolognaise for dinner and we sat and
ate while she and Leo told tales of their day. I listened intently,

thinking about the diary entries I had read earlier on. I had so many questions yet was afraid of hearing the answers. After dinner and some light TV (I was adjusting slowly), Leo went for his nightly bath while Simone and I washed the dishes. I told her about the diary entries I had read and questioned her about the drugs. She explained that Adult Naomi had started to smoke weed from around sixteen but even when the craving was great, she had never smoked around Leo. Simone didn't like it when she smoked, as she always saw Adult Naomi's life taking a turn for the worse when she did. She wouldn't sleep or eat properly and she would eventually slip into deep depressions. She then started doing cocaine when she moved into her big house and met Sasha and Noelle. I didn't know who she was talking about and felt nothing when she said their names.

'Lovely women, but shallow,' Simone stated.

'Shallow?' What was she on about?

'Yeah, lots of money, big cars, bigger houses. But no amount of money or designer clothes can substitute for a life of substance, Nay.'

'Yeah, like, shame. Even I know that,' I said.

Simone explained that Adult Naomi had gone through a lot in that house. When Leo was three she finished working for the haulage company and tried the Chinese medicine degree. She didn't like that so she went to college and did a diploma in alternative therapies instead. She then set her own business up with some money from the Prince's Trust when she was twenty-six and moved into this 'big house' when she was twenty-seven. Adult Naomi was earning good money and hanging around with friends who were also living the champagne and cocaine lifestyle. It made me think of that comedy *Absolutely Fabulous*, except this was far from funny. Simone told me that she was a highly sought-after healer and teacher of holistic therapies, and that she had also developed and sold her own cosmetics. And she was at university doing her psychology degree.

So she *was* trying to build an empire! Cool.

This lifestyle had apparently been her downfall so she had moved to Greece to live with Marlene. This hadn't worked out so she came home and ended up homeless in a hostel, still taking drugs, trying to get her life together.

The entry I had read from the 2006 diary was written the night she moved into the hostel. The other entry was from her 2007 diary and was the last time she ever did cocaine. Simone informed me that Adult Naomi and Sasha did a load of pure-cut Columbian cocaine one night and she vowed she would never take another line of coke unless she was actually in Columbia itself.

Exsqueeze me?

Judging from the 2008 diary, she hadn't continued, but I was still totally grossed out that she had even started down that path. Simone said the diaries would explain more and that I needed to read them to find out why she had made the choices she had. I silently dried the dishes as I listened to her try and fill in the blanks. It was difficult for her because there had been long periods of time when Adult Naomi hadn't spoken to her and she hadn't known what was going on in her life.

'I know. I was, like, seriously raging at you at times. Our relationship has been majorly messed up, hasn't it, Sim?'

'Hmm.' She nodded and sighed. 'Sometimes, and then sometimes it's been great, but we've tried, Nay. We have been on our own from a young age, you know.'

'Sim, what's with me analysing my problems all the time? God, it can send you all a bit mental.'

She laughed and dried her hands. 'Before you lost your memory, you were doing a self-empowerment class for women. You were really trying to get your life back together. Erm, and, well, girl, you've always been deep, a thinker; it's the psychologist in you, and the weed.'

'Yeah, but even I know that's just, like, a bad combination, you know?' I placed the dried dishes in the cupboard.

'Oh yeah, it's definitely been to your own detriment some-times.' She looked at me, troubled. 'I mean, you've been that stressed, you've lost your memory and you're trying to deal with it all by yourself.'

'Well, it's got to bloody stop.' I threw down the tea towel. 'Naaa, maaan, this is, like, complete PANTS! I need to stop the drugs and smoking, this body needs some serious exer-cise, and, you know, to be a bit more healthy, and all this analysing is *sooooo saaaad,* and going for men who are like Dad or Joseph . . . ugh, gross Mr Morose.' I stuck my fingers down my throat in mock throw-up fashion. 'I mean, forget boys, woman, sort your sad smeggin' life out!'

Simone chuckled. 'Never did get the dad thing, but it's a plan and I like plans!'

'And I'm going to help her sort it out, starting by going through those bloody diaries . . . The hostel one was so sad.' I could feel the lump again.

'I know, we didn't speak for months when you were in

there, but I'm here for you if you need anything, sis, and I'm really proud of you.' Simone gave me a strong and loving hug.

We weren't very affectionate with each other usually – she wouldn't stop using my hair gel – and sometimes our fights rivalled Ali and Foreman's jungle rumble. But here, now, it felt good when she hugged me.

I told Simone to leave that night when Leo was safe and sound in bed. She didn't want to, but I reassured her I would be fine again until she came back the next day.

I had had enough of TV, so sat in the bedroom and forced myself to go back to the diaries.

28 May 2006

The end of an era. Well, the end of me living in this house for now anyway. Moving is horrible; well, it has been this time, you know, really has, but there's nothing to keep me here. I have to go. The tears, the sheer sadness of saying goodbye to my personal belongings. Letting go of the material things is really hard – really hard; so many memories attached to them, people, places, and things. Watching those objects of comfort, the bed, the sofa, even the Sky box, being moved elsewhere, it has been more difficult than I anticipated. I didn't realize how attached to everything I am and for a moment I wanted to scream to the removal man to put it all back, that I have changed my mind. But I can't go back, I know I can't; I have no choice, no option. I have to move on. But I am allowed to be sad about it. Just need to wait now, wait for the medication to kick in and things will get better.

This confirmed what Simone had told me earlier. Adult Naomi had moved from her last house voluntarily, but felt like she had no choice. Why? And what medication was she taking?

I flipped backwards through the pages to three months before she left the house.

13 February 2006

Feeling my way through the darkness, I think I can see a light at the end of the tunnel. Not sure whether to trust it, but maybe in the end I have no choice but to surrender to it. Nothing makes sense, yet it all does at the same time; I'm living the paradox, existing somewhere in between the two realities. Simple decisions are mammoth choices, easy tasks become complex puzzles for me to figure my way through, and sad songs bring me peace, a sense of calm, and then I cry. If I think too much, my brain flips to thinking crazy, manic thoughts; I imagine I can save the world, that I am a god, that nobody understands the patterns, the signs, and then I get high trying to stop the waterfalls in my mind. Can't control those thoughts from falling, crashing, smacking, banging into my brain. Smack smack smack! Still no sleep, still cry; every day I cry, cry, cry; it feels like it will never end. Do you cry when you die?

And that's all I know right now, isn't it? Death. Will I be like the caterpillar and transform into a butterfly? Or will my chrysalis, devoid of providence, wither up and die?

Will I become a former shell of the beauty I once was? Live without the sparkle? Light? Warmth? Safety? Just be?

But was I ever? Or is that just a dream? Or has it always been like this? So painful, so confusing, so scary, without love.

Love? The meaning of this word escapes the grasp of my comprehension.

I had a thought today while I was driving: it's not that I hate myself; I just haven't found a reason to love myself. I'm sure there was a time I used to at least like myself for being different, for not being like everyone else. And then I tried to be like everyone else and I ended up very unhappy, and after being around those I tried to be like, I realized they were deeply unhappy. And they didn't have the answers I was searching for. They have just accepted it as their lot. Am I now accepting it as my lot? The concept of liking myself got lost in the fog, and I can't seem to find it. Faraway yet so close. Somewhere deep down inside of me, I know I can find it, but there's this great fear; I have to leave, I know I do. I need to be patient, I need to be brave and pray this week gets better and not worse, just better; better in the sense that it all makes sense again, and you know what, I think it will.

N xxx

Obviously, it so didn't. I went back one week previous.

? February 2006 (forgot the date, thinks it's the fifth or sixth, but who cares)

I'm stuck, stuck fast and ain't budging. Fear causes paralysis and right now I'm comfortably numb, telling myself I cannot for the love of God move. I'm tired, fed

*up, stoned and miserable. I wanna cry over everything
and nothing, but mainly over the fact that I am stuck. It's
snowing outside, all white and harmless looking, except
really it's bloody freezing and can kill you with its zero
below fire. I've had enough of the snow. I've had enough
of this life. I AM TIRED!! And so full of hate, and anger;
it has nowhere to go but right back into despair and then
I'm numb again. I am comfort eating like it's going out of
fashion; even getting high is exasperating me only because
I don't know if I am or not!? Uni's shagged; I have fallen
so far behind with my work and to top it all – wahey! –
I've been diagnosed with bipolar disorder! Is this the
outcome of my mother's love?*

Where did I go?

Where's my strength gone?

WAS I EVER HERE?

WAS IT EVER HERE?

*My determination, my will to live, to live life to the
fullest, is elusive.*

*I still believe somewhere I did something terribly
wrong, that I deserve this, that I deserve to feel this way.
All's I want to do is hide away. Hide away and never
come out again. It hurts too much. It's too painful.*

Hold up. Wait a minute! What the hell is bipolar disorder?
I placed the diaries down and called Katie. She answered
on the second ring.

'Hiya, babe. How are you feeling?'

'Do you know what bipolar is?'

'What?'

'Tell me it's got something to do with ice caps, snow and chaotic bears.'

She laughed. 'What? No, why do you want to know, love?'

'It's okay, I'm okay. I've been reading the diaries.'

'Oh, right.' Katie took a deep breath. 'You've had a bad time of it, Nay, and you ended up having a breakdown.'

'A breakdown?'

'Yes, babe. You went through a lot of bad things, and at the time, you couldn't cope. So in the end, you went to a psychiatrist and they diagnosed you with bipolar disorder.'

'But what is it? What happened to me?'

'It used to be called manic depression, like when people get severe mood swings. Sometimes you'd be high for days; you wouldn't sleep or eat and you'd have loads of energy. And then sometimes you'd be low, really low, and would stay in bed for days, weeks, depressed and crying.'

'Wow.'

'Yeah, it was really bad at one point, but you sorted yourself out; things got better, you went on medication, you moved to Greece, you tried a different life.'

'Yeah, and ended up homeless.' I didn't mention the drugs; I felt too ashamed.

'Oh no, babe, that was stuff that you couldn't control. You didn't know what would happen when you went to Greece.'

I went quiet. I didn't want to know.

'So, what causes it then? Why did I get it?'

'I'm not sure, hun. I think some people say it's genetic; others have said it's drug use, or stuff from your childhood looking for a way to get out. I think with you it was lots of things, all happening at once.'

'Oh, okay.' It suddenly came to me – *the boo boo*; was bipolar the boo boo?

'So what happened then? Does she . . . I mean, do I still have it? Should I be taking medication now?' I thought about Doctor Davies, eager to give me the sleeping tablets. Was he just trying to knock the bipolar out?

'What? No,' Katie insisted. 'Not at all. You've gone a long time without them now. You didn't want to become dependent on them; you started to take alternative remedies, do you remember?'

I didn't, but felt a bit better hearing Adult Naomi was trying to control it somehow.

'You've been really strong, Nay, you really have. You've been through a lot of stress, but you're still here.'

Except she wasn't. Adult Naomi had left the bloody building, leaving me to find out that before she went she was in a really tapped mental tossing place. I felt ashamed at first, as this was majorly, majorly rank, and then got angry with her. How could she let things get so bad that she had to see a psychiatrist? Bipolar disorder! But there it was, just like with transient global amnesia, that frickin' word again: STRESS!

My head started to feel dizzy. I was stepping into territory I didn't understand and didn't have a clue how to navigate, but I wanted to carry on. I needed to get to the bottom of this stress. A strange feeling was beginning to creep up on me, suggesting that all of this had something to do with why I had now appeared in her life at this exact point. I sighed deeply.

'Are you okay, Nay? Do you want me to come round for a cuppa? I can be there in five minutes.'

At that moment, Katie's warm, smiling, calming energy

sounded comforting, but I wanted to carry on. I needed to know more.

'No, I'm okay right now; maybe tomorrow,' I whispered, trying to sound as grateful as possible.

'Okay, love, but I want you to remember something, Nay. You are really strong and brave and everything you did in life, you did because you wanted to live a better life for you and Leo.'

'Okay.' I wasn't convinced; to me, drugs were not a way to live a better life. 'I'm gonna go now, get a bath, go to bed.'

'Right. Call me if you need me.'

'I will. Thanks, Katie.'

'Any time, love, bye-dee-bye,' she sang.

'Bye.' I smiled and hung up the phone.

I picked the diary up and continued.

7

Remember Me

Forget me not
My flower.
Forget me not
My dear.
Forget me not
My love.

R. W.

7 January 2006

I can smell the stench of death beckoning me.
   Is there peace in the chaos?
   Peace in death?
   Death.
   Maybe I should give in to it, maybe it's the only way.
I look at the razor blades every time I walk into the
bathroom; one slice and it's over.
   Yes.
   Death.

I let out a cry. Death? Why was everything so dark, and her only way out was suicide? What about Leo? What about Simone? Didn't they matter to her? What could have possibly happened to her to get her to this place of despair? Each entry I read just seemed to get worse; she had spiralled into depression, a helter-skelter ride of sad saddo despairishness.

I closed the diary. I had no choice but to let it out, caving into the pull of deep sorrow. It seemed to bind with the same suffering in the pages. Poor Adult Naomi, she was in a bad way, she was so full of hopelessness that even the thought of leaving Leo seemed like a better option than staying and subjecting him to her fear and sorrow.

I couldn't see any more words on the page for the flood of tears flowing from my eyes. I needed to cry for her. I lay my head on the pillow. Maybe, I thought, deep down she was still feeling the same way, maybe it's why she still took cocaine and smoked weed, maybe this was why she had never decorated her bedroom, and maybe it was why I had turned up. Maybe.

I turned over and cried myself into a deep sleep. My only thought was how terribly sorry I felt for Adult Naomi. This wasn't the way things were supposed to be. This wasn't a good future.

I woke up the next day to sounds of Leo flushing the toilet. Thoughts of him and his smiling face gave me the energy to jump out of bed. I took one look in the mirror and remembered what I had read the night before. My face was swollen, my eyes puffy. I smiled anyway because I wanted Leo to see – no, feel – that everything was okay. I shouted good morning to him and made my way downstairs, stopping for a second to

look again at the photos on the wall. They were full of glowing smiles. Adult Naomi looked so happy; she must have been
once. Leo looked so content. Why had those smiles stopped? I
still had so much to find out.

I made Leo breakfast and while we ate he told me about a
boy who used to be his friend, but since he had started skating
he wasn't his friend any more.

'He said that I think I'm the best at skating and he said
I'm not, but I don't, Mum. I just practise more than him,' he
protested.

'Well, what did you say to him?' I asked, wondering what
was the right thing to tell a ten-year-old boy how to handle
other kids of the same age.

'I told him to build a bridge and get over it.' He bit into his
pancake.

I burst out laughing and almost spilt my herbal tea all over
myself. Leo laughed as well.

'You're the bees, Leo Jacobs.' I patted him on the back and
then followed him as he grabbed his coat and bag and disappeared through the front door.

I was grateful Adult Naomi had held on to him and held
on to her life. This little boy deserved the best that life had
to offer, including a loving mother. Which, judging by his
wicked personality and funny bones, he had had through
his little life.

When he left, I thought about what he had said: *build a
bridge and get over it*. Maybe that's what I needed to do, build
some sort of mental bridge from me to Adult Naomi, and get
over it. Somehow get to the other side. Maybe then I would
get into the house in my mind and find her.

I ran a bath and while I waited for it to fill, I opened the diary at a random page. It was seven months before the 'depressive downer darkness' had descended.

16 June 2005

Okay, so there's much more balance in my existence and its feels buena! *Cooked a lovely dinner – another good thing about me, I am a great cook! Everyone ate their dinner; they've all gone to the park and the house is quiet. I'm lying on my bed writing this. Karl has just left. I saved him some dinner; he ate it all while providing me with light conversation and jokes. I'm feeling very peaceful. I'm glad he took me up on my offer to come for dinner; it was nice and I'm in a much better place concerning our relationship. I am happy and content just being friends with him. Is this contentment? Cooking for my family and friends? If so, then I'll do it more definitely. I love that I'm clearing things out. Three things I like about myself today: I am a good friend, a good mum and a good cook. I've got great friends in my life, work is going well – busier than I have ever been – and, well, I think I'll be okay for my exams also. Think I'll read my book for a while.*

Naomi x

So things were okay with Adult Naomi sometimes. I didn't understand why she had needed to find things to like about herself; surely she already knew she was a good person. She was friends with her ex. She was surrounded by family and enjoyed cooking.

My curiosity about what had happened in the time in

between the okay times and the traumatic times, hung on a thin line, like a photograph slowly developing, but now I wanted to know about her spars. Where the hell were they when all this happened? Why did it only seem to be Simone and Katie? Where were Eve and Art? And where the hell was Leo's father in all of this?

I was beginning to feel desperate for answers.

I spent the rest of the day reading more diary entries, mainly the ones that came after Adult Naomi was told she had bipolar and had lost the house she loved so much. From 2006 to 2008, her words in the pages gave me more of an explanation.

It seemed that the best option for her had been to quit university, and because she had fallen into debt, move in with Simone while she was on medication and wait until Leo had finished his primary school year. It provided her with some stability and normalcy. During the summer of 2006, she had moved to Greece to live with my stepmum Marlene (Art's exgirlfriend) and her Greek husband. Turns out Adult Naomi had gone from the frying pan into the Mediterranean fire. Marlene was a heavy drinker and after Adult Naomi confronted her over it, they had a blazing row and she and Leo left, finding themselves homeless and stranded in Greece.

At the end of that summer, she moved back to England, tried to live with Simone – it didn't work out as they had a blazing row (*Are you frickin' kidding me?*) – and then she put herself and Leo in a hostel in the autumn whilst attempting to finish her last year at uni. Seven months later, in 2007, she was offered a house, this house.

A year later, in April 2008, I turned up.

This brought me up to speed, but it was what had happened in the year between her being 'a great cook' and being bipolar that I needed to know about.

Reading the rest of the entries took up most of my day. I'd become curious about the people in Adult Naomi's life and when Simone came back from work – carrying pizzas – I told her of my plans to go and see Adult Naomi's friends at some point. She thought it was a good idea. Maybe it would help me remember.

Wrapped in a protective bubble created by Simone and Katie, I stayed locked away in the small two-bedroom house and spent days getting lost in the world of an adult I didn't quite understand, yet felt well sorry for. I tucked away the diary I'd nicknamed the '3Ds' – downer, depressive, darkness – not yet quite ready to delve back into that world, at least not until I had met Adult Naomi's friends.

I slipped comfortably into a routine of seeing Leo off to school, curling up on the sofa, and reading the pre-'3Ds' entries. Her large collection of DVDs broke up the day, as unless it was 1990s programming, my brain couldn't cope with regular television; it still all seemed so fake, so unreal. I survived on beans on toast, fruit, tuna fish sandwiches, and jacket potatoes zapped in the microwave and laden with cottage cheese.

The diaries were in chronological order, so I worked my way backwards from 2008 to 1995. There was a two-year gap between 1993 and 1994 where she didn't write at all. I worked out that it was when she was seventeen, eighteen and nineteen. I asked Simone what happened to her then. She said it had a lot to do with LSD and magic mushrooms. Yeah, Adult Naomi had taken this hippie trippy thing way too far.

Still, I read on. Each diary had about eighteen months' to two years' of her personal thoughts and her innermost secrets. Some of it was fascinating; some of it was horrifying; some of it was a bit tapped at times. Some I thought was hilarious and some of it was really sad – not saddo sad, but, like, unhappy sad.

There were times I had to put the book I was reading down and breathe deeply. These were her memories, her beliefs, and her experiences of a world as she saw it. Stuff about the people she had chosen to be around, the relationships she had, the jobs she had worked in, and the men she had tried to love. While reading it I kind of hoped it would bring back some memories, or I would get a feeling of déjà vu, but nothing happened. It was like I was reading all these different stories and they made up a book of someone else's life.

In the evening, Simone and Katie sorted me and Leo out with dinner and distraction. Leo was oblivious, which I thought was cool; it must have meant that he felt safe with me. His year-six homework was a cinch, although I was confused over the whole Americanization thing again, asking Simone when it had stopped being fourth-year juniors.

We also played lots of his wicked Xbox and Wii games when Simone had to work late or when he didn't wanna leave our house because it was raining outside.

Each day was like some weird *Quantum Leap* episode. I wanted so badly to remember and figure some things out, all the time scared of what I would find.

Adult Naomi's diaries told me how she had met Leo's father

and what, after promising herself she would never have children, had led her to be a mother at twenty-one. She used to have this, like, saddo desperate need to be loved by him and he was a bit of a div to her. In fact, no, a total tosspotting smeghead at times. She had found out he had been cheating on her when she was eight months pregnant and she broke it off with him. It also felt like a constant battle to get him to spend time with Leo outside of the six hours every other Sunday he seemed to think was enough. He wasn't there for parents' evenings or Leo's extra-curricular activities, and she'd get stressed on Sundays because he wouldn't call if he was running late or wasn't able to come at all. He also didn't offer to help out with extra expenses for Leo, thinking twenty pounds a week for maintenance was sufficient. And when Leo was four years old, he told her he never wanted to spend time with Leo on his own because it made him feel guilty about his other three children.

Even I knew, at fifteen, that was complete and utter pants. The mentalism of it all was that Adult Naomi couldn't see it. In one of her diary entries she wrote, 'I know I have in the past tried to force him, bribe him, persuade him, love and hate him into being a proper father to Leo and nothing has worked – it may be that nothing will ever work – but I am not going to stop trying.'

He even had the complete crapness to attack her mind whenever she caught him in a lie, calling her crazy and mental. I read that they argued while she was in the hostel the night after she had confided in him about the bipolar-bear mentalism and losing her home. He had gone to the gym instead of picking Leo up. Why hadn't he offered her and Leo a place to stay? I just found myself getting angrier and angrier the more I read about him and decided that he wasn't worth my time or energy. I so far hadn't met him since waking up in the future and, going from what I had read, I *sooooo* didn't want to.

But after calming down, I realized that as much as her choice in father had been a mistake, having Leo was not and never would be a mistake. He was too kriss biscuits* of a child to ever regret, and besides, it seemed Adult Naomi had done a good enough job without him anyway.

I moved on.

I read about the friends she had made over the years; some long gone, others still around. It seemed she forgave people but didn't forget, and was really loyal to the peeps she loved. Even when these so-called spars lied to her, used her, and totally Jekylled** her.

Eventually, she just seemed to give herself a hard time and kept promising that she would learn her lesson from every experience or mistake so as not to repeat it again. *Exsqueeze me?* I thought. *Even I know it ain't totally your fault when someone is acting like a complete wackass and you don't see it coming! Why would you blame yourself for people's mental tosser issues?*

Adult Naomi had analysed and dissected and picked apart her experiences over and over, read self-help book after self-help book, attended empowerment classes, workshops, and therapy sessions. I was exhausted just reading about it. She

---

* *Kriss biscuits* – really really gorgeous and fabulous and lovely and great and cute and all the brilliant words you can think of wrapped in a chocolate biscuit!
** *Jekyll* – two-faced/very deceitful.

had, like, this desperate need to figure out her 'motivations', to 'transform', to continually force herself to 'change and grow'. She was always worrying about the effect the past had on her and how it was going to affect her future.

In my opinion, she was demonstrating severe Molecule-Mind saddo behaviour. Which made her find comfort in mood-altering drugs, therapy, films and books. It also seemed she had a slight addiction to painkillers and every now and then she would quit the weed just so she could convince herself she wasn't an addict. It seemed like being addicted to something was the only way Adult Naomi felt she could control stuff that had seriously damaged her mind mojo.

Her relationship with Simone was very close, but they lived on the opposite sides of the city because most times they ended up becoming what she called 'co-dependently' close. She said they had 'boundary issues'.

After running away and marrying the postman (*seriously?*), my mum, Eve, would visit once a year. She lived in London and her drinking seemed to, like, mash everything up. Adult Naomi put it like this: 'Seeing Eve is like holding up a mirror to everything dysfunctional that existed in our childhoods.' So, by the age of thirty-two, Adult Naomi had not spoken to Eve properly in four years. I wasn't exactly surprised, but I needed to know what had happened. Maybe her friends would help me.

Dean. He was the first of Adult Naomi's friends I contacted.

I had read in the 1995 diary that when she was nineteen she had moved to Manchester to live with the daughter of a Scottish-Jewish family called the Goldfeins. It didn't say why she had moved to Manchester and the daughter was no longer in Adult Naomi's life (this seemed to happen a lot with her girlfriends, I noticed), but Dean, whom she had met at the same time, was.

From her journal entries, I could tell that her relationship with him was very important and she well loved him, like a friend or a big brother.

While reading the diary entries, I got a nice déjà vu every time he was mentioned and he always seemed to make her laugh and tell her really wack jokes, which she found hilarious. When she was with Dean, she laughed until her stomach hurt, so I liked the sound of him.

He seemed like a safe, chilled guy and when I finished reading about him, I imagined him lying on one of those narrow boats with one foot in the cool water, floating downstream, chewing on a blade of straw, the sunshine on his smiling face, not knowing where he was going, but flowing with it nonetheless. When she had told him her problems, he was totally real with her, told her straight, and left her with what she called a 'Deanism'.

When I read his last words to her before she left the building, I knew I wanted to speak to him. Those words were, 'Sis, it's just a hump and you'll get over it.'

That evening, I found his number and called him while Simone was helping Leo with his homework.

Having not spoken for weeks, he was pleased to hear from me. He went silent when I had to explain to him why.

'Wow, sis, that's some serious stuff.' He had a really strong Manchester accent.

'I know . . . I mean, I know I know you . . . but I don't remember you.'

'Awesome. Far out. What a trip,' he said slowly.

'I know, but Sim's looking after me and Leo's *sooooo* cool.'

'Wow, this is as rare as rocking-horse shit.' He paused and his voice went an octave higher. '*Don't take the brown acid,*' he mocked in a strange American accent.

I didn't know jack about what he was talking about, but his laugh made me wanna laugh.

'I know!' I chuckled.

For the first time, I could see from someone else's point of view that there possibly could be a funny side to losing your memory. It *was* far out; it *was* the stuff of science fiction movies and bad acid Woodstock experiences (he explained about Wavy Gravy). It was also fascinating and awesome and scarily funny. I mean, who does this really happen to? Who gets so stressed that they actually lose their memory?

'Sis, you've gotta chill the fuck out, seriously,' Dean said. 'You know what? Fuck the world and just do what you wanna do for real. It's time for Naomi to take care of Naomi. You can't keep getting stressed out like this.'

I so agreed. Adult Naomi had taken herself way too seriously for too long and then beaten herself up constantly over other people's tosserness. I mean, she had never intentionally harmed anyone; nobody had died, so why in a world full of such crap and confusion had she made her life more miserable with this mega dumping truck of guilt? No wonder she had someone like Dean in her life; she needed him.

We carried on talking for another five minutes, but I had to end the conversation when my head started to hurt because I was trying too hard to remember him.

He was safe, though, well funny, and I said goodbye to him with my sense of humour sorted. If Adult Naomi didn't come back, I knew I would definitely keep him in my life no matter what.

One of her other close friends was on a cruise ship somewhere deep in the Pacific Ocean and was incommunicado. Her name was Georgina and I liked the sound of her in the diaries and was interested to meet her when she got back to the UK. The same could not be said for her other spars, though. I didn't quite understand the friendships. But if I wanted answers, I had to meet them.

A couple of Saturdays later, on a bright, warm day – Leo was with Simone overnight – I decided it was time for me to brave the outside world and find my way to Adult Naomi's other friends.

I could still remember how to drive, but wasn't confident enough to put my fifteen-year-old self behind a wheel. Simone had given me directions and the numbers of the buses and trams I needed to take. I nearly fell backwards through the set of doors on the futuristic bus when the driver told me how much it would cost to get to the city centre. I'd never been on a tram before so it was a bit of a novelty to ride on one when I got to the city. It was rickety and bounced you around a bit, but it helped me see a little more of Manchester.

Manchester. I had only ever been to Manchester once. My dad had taken me when I was thirteen and my uncle Jack got married to his new wife, and I remembered how my aunties had kept sniggering and whispering that his new father-in-law looked like Uncle Fester from the Addams Family.

It looked so different now. There were lots of factories and cotton mills that had been turned into apartments sitting next to old valleys densely filled with trees and spring flowers. The canal was lined with bars, clubs and shops. Brand-new apartment buildings and offices, and a large shopping centre, towered over the hundreds of people coming and going.

I sat on the tram watching Adult Naomi's world fly by until a man sitting opposite me smiled. 'I knew it was going to be you,' he said. *Is he talking to me?* I thought. *Oh crap, does he know Adult Naomi?* I turned around to make sure he wasn't talking to anyone behind me. His eyes had a strange glassy stare, so I gave him a half-smile. 'I'm sorry, I . . . I don't remem—' I stammered.

'I know,' he replied. 'I've had so much work on. It's been too long; we are due a drink, darling.' He shifted in his seat, looked the other way, and carried on talking.

There was a five-second delay and then I realized he wasn't talking to me; he was in fact talking to his headphones, which must have been connected to his hidden mobile phone.

I'd seen this when I was in Simone's car driving along the streets of the village. At first, when I had noticed people walking, talking and laughing to themselves, I'd assumed they were bonkers. Like Loopy Larry, our town 'crazy' who walked around unshaven, with tired yellowing eyes and grey hair, asking, 'Do you have a penny, missus?' every time he saw you. We would tease him as kids and run away from him, laughing. But one day, Eve told me what had turned him crazy. He was highly intelligent and had a psychology degree but when his brother died he suffered a heavy mental breakdown, from which he had never recovered. I never laughed at him again . . . Simone explained that Adult Naomi hadn't actually moved to a city full of Larrys and told me about hands-free mobile technology.

This explained why nobody on the tram batted an eyelid when a random stranger started to talk to himself. But seriously, in a world of Bluetooth, how do you separate the sane from the crazy if everyone is walking around talking to themselves? And what was with the headphones? It seemed every other person had a pair stuck in their ears and escaped into a world of downloaded music; everyone in their own worlds, like the new social networking stuff, was making people severely antisocial.

One thing I did notice, though, was old people were still open to the world around them. When I made eye contact with a foge* on the bus or on the tram, they smiled at me, they made a comment, they even sparked up a conversation about the weather. They weren't afraid to talk to me. I mean, even I knew sometimes it was good to talk to a random stranger – so long as you weren't on your own and the stranger wasn't a man in a red cap. For a second, I wondered why I always imagined crazed serial killers wearing red caps and then, as I noticed a white-haired woman in her sixties watching the world go by, I kinda hoped all the old people in the world stuck around for a little bit longer, just so people didn't forget how to talk to each other.

The city centre was manic and as I stepped off the tram I

---

* *Foge/old fogey* – a kind, elderly person.

almost got swept away in a sea of people. It was overwhelming and my head started to hurt as soon as I tried to think where to go, so I sat on the metal bench at the station, trying to get my thoughts together. There were young mothers pushing strange-looking tiny prams with three massive wheels past people laden with shopping bags. I didn't know if it was possible but the Goths standing outside a rock music shop seemed to look more serious and stand with more of a hunch. I mean, after black, there's not really any other way to go, but I swear their clothes looked blacker, their eyeliner thicker and their hair greasier. I wondered if those were the emos, the new Goths Simone had told me about? She'd also told me that the Farrah-trouser-V-neck-jumper-wearing crew (usually with no shirt and a gold chain on their hairless chest) had been replaced by Burberry-cap-wearing-tracksuit-clad 'chavs' with silver chains around their necks.

I studied the shop windows; they were full of the bizarro 'embellished' bags, shoes and jackets covered with metallic gold and silver studs I had seen in the magazines. The mannequins had no faces, and were again dressed in the weird coloured fashions I had seen in Adult Naomi's wardrobe. Primark, All Saints, H&M, Zara, Mango, American Apparel; bandage, boho, rock, girly, country chic. So many different stores, so many different styles and so much choice; how did you know where to go? It had to be confusing to know which style to choose and which shops to shop in, which look was yours. How did you keep up? Where was C&A?

After studying the people and the shops for a while, my brain seemed to settle into a quiet buzz. It was then that I noticed the coffee shops, four of them in my three-hundred-

and-sixty-degree sight, all walking distance from each other. Costa, Starbucks (wasn't that a character from *Battlestar Galactica*?) Nero and Coffee Hut! Why was there so much need for coffee? When did Britain become a nation of coffee lovers? What had happened to Mr Tetley?

I was curious – maybe this was why Adult Naomi was ser-iously into coffee – so I made my way to the nearest one. It was mega busy. I stood in the queue, feeling mesmerized by all of the cakes on offer, the sandwiches, the breakfast rolls. When I looked up at the boards behind the counter my jaw almost hit the floor. There was a list of coffees as long as the eighteen-metre bus I had just ridden on. I had a coffee conundrum. All this choice again.

Eventually, I saw the more familiar hot chocolate and settled on that. While I waited, the woman behind the cash register served the man stood in front of me.

'What can I get you, sir?' she asked.

'I'll have a medio non-fat double decaf latte, medio soya milk mocha with cinnamon and a grande americano with vanilla to go.'

I watched the woman touch the screen. It was just like the phone – no buttons again. She repeated his order. She didn't even tell him how much; he just put his cash card in the little machine and punched in a few numbers. They didn't exchange another word.

'What can I get you?' She looked straight at me.

'Erm.' I turned to her and then looked at the board. 'Err, a hot chocolate, please.'

'One hot chocolate; stay in or take out?'

'Err . . . in?' I asked her.

'Anything else?'

'Err . . . no.' I was relieved to hear at least this drink was still the same.

'Do you want full-fat, half-fat or non-fat milk, or soya?'

'Full-fat?' I took a guess.

She pressed on the screen again without saying a word. 'Do you want whipped cream and marshmallows?'

'Oh, yeah.' I smiled.

She repeated my order. I then nearly fell face first into the biscotti when she told me my drink would cost almost a fiver! *FIVE POUNDS!* For a hot chocolate! *Are you kidding me?* I wanted to ask her. *Is this, like, a joke?* First the magazines, then the bus fare, and now this?

But I could tell by the impatient look on her face that she wasn't joking. I gave her a dirty look (like inflation was her fault) but she didn't notice, took my money, and shouted, 'Next!' I took this as my cue to move on; no small talk, no friendly banter. Again, it was the same weird, detached feeling I'd felt in the supermarket. All of a sudden, buying a hot chocolate seemed a lonely affair. I didn't let it stop me, though. I thought of the old foges on the bus.

'Like a Christmas list,' I joked to the coffee-making guy. 'Never seen so much coffee in one place.' I nodded at the list on the wall.

He looked puzzled, gave a half-smile, and started to bang this metal thing around loudly. Nobody took any notice, so I assumed this meant the banging was normal and he wasn't actually threatening to off me with coffee-making implements.

He poured my drink into a glass (a glass!), squirted cream

on top, and sprinkled it with tiny pink and white marsh-mallows.

I sat down at a small table by the window and stared at my drink as if it was an expensive piece of art. I felt like I had to – it had cost me a frickin' fiver!

As I slowly sipped my chocolate, I watched the people in the coffee shop. A Muslim family came over and sat at the table next to me. As the young woman took her baby out of its buggy she smiled at me. I smiled back, and the little girl looked over at me and giggled. She was total cuteness with curly hair and big brown eyes. I mock giggled back and she buried her face into her mother's chest. The man gave a friendly smile and I went back to my chocolate, but not before noticing a couple on the other side of them shuffling their seats slightly away, eyeing them suspiciously. *Are you kidding me?* I thought. *What, are people, like, thinking all Muslims are bad, as if this friendly family are smuggling weapons of mass destruction in a baby's nappy? Jeez Louise!*

Happy that the world still had some friendly people in it, despite other people's ignorance, I finished my arty chocolate. It was time to find my way to Maeve's house.

Maeve seemed nice. She was tall and skinny with straight blonde hair and sharp green eyes. She made us both a hot drink, sat at the kitchen table, and rolled a joint. It took me five minutes to realize this woman was deeply unhappy. She reminded me of a character called Sad Sack from *The Raggy Dolls* cartoon, dolls that nobody wanted, who lived in the reject bin. Sad Sack was perpetually miserable and always looked on the negative side of life. To him, existence was doomed and there was no point in doing anything because all effort was futile.

The more I studied her face, the more I realized she looked older than she was and had experienced way too much in her life, including an abusive partner who had a drink problem and hit her on a regular basis over the years. She had tried to leave him on many occasions, sometimes even turning up at Adult Naomi's with a black eye or two, but in the end, she always went back to him. This was all in the diaries and Simone had told me some of it as well.

It was difficult to hide the being a fifteen-year-old thing from Maeve, but she was too stoned to see anything was different and I managed to get a few details from her with regards what had happened to Adult Naomi after the June 2005 diary entry when everything seemed okay. She smoked joint after joint and cigarette after cigarette, and drank coffee after coffee, while reminding me of the car accident that Adult Naomi had been involved in in the summer of 2005 which had left her with severe whiplash. She'd ignored the warnings the doctor had given her and gone horse riding, where she'd got thrown off a giant horse and broken two ribs. She wasn't able to work for more than a year and she started to lose money and get into debt. Maybe this was how she had lost her house.

As she talked on, I'd had enough. I had to leave before the mushroom cloud of smoke Maeve existed in threatened to wipe me off the planet. I chipped as soon as possible.

As I took a taxi to Danielle's, Adult Naomi's other friend, I wondered what had happened to Katie, my real best friend from school. I hadn't found her in the diaries – or this future life – yet.

Danielle seemed happy to see me, saying, 'It's been too long,' when she hugged me.

She was around the same height as me, had the same complexion, but was slimmer with shorter hair. I liked her immediately, until she rolled a joint. I was starting to see a pattern here and wasn't happy. She had a daughter around the same age as Leo and Adult Naomi had known her and her family since she was pregnant. From the diaries, I knew that Danielle was like family to her and there had been many tough times when they had relied on each other as they were both single mothers with unreliable men for fathers. Adult Naomi had found Danielle hilarious, like, stand-up-comic hilarious, especially when she'd had a drink. But like family, they had had problems and disagreements as well. Still, like with Dean, I got a good feeling of déjà vu when I was around her, a kind of comfortableness you only get when you're with family. I knew it was okay to take my shoes off and relax on the sofa with the cup of herbal tea she'd made for me. It was so different from Maeve's. The mood was lighter, less intense. I told her of the stress Katie and Simone told me that Adult Naomi had experienced before the memory loss, but stopped before the break-up with 'French Dude'. Thankfully, she didn't know much about him, but we spoke about men and I was glad to hear she had left a relationship that she knew was no longer good for her. Something she had realized since the death of 'our friend'.

I tried to get as much information as possible from her about this friend when I realized this was again before the

'3Ds' diary period in Adult Naomi's life. It was like piecing together a picture puzzle of a quiet storm and these were the corner pieces, the edges of the black clouds.

'Beautiful' (my nickname for her) was a mutual friend who'd died of breast cancer. Adult Naomi had grown close to her during her treatment, and they used to go for power walks and had even decided to go into business together before she grew too ill. But she had died, devastating everyone who knew her and the two children she had left behind. She had obviously had a big effect on Adult Naomi's life because she'd been too upset to go to the funeral.

Danielle stopped talking about her halfway through the conversation; I could see it was still too painful for her, so I didn't push. Instead, I finished my tea and asked her to call me a taxi.

I left feeling sad and a little bit confused about Danielle. She and Adult Naomi obviously had a history, but apart from being single parents, smoking weed and having the odd drink together, I couldn't see what exactly they had in common and whether what they had was enough.

Next I wanted to meet Rhonda, the second closest friend in Adult Naomi's life, the woman she had gone to Paris with before Adult Naomi disappeared and whose description in her diaries left me slightly confused. On the one hand, Adult Naomi loved her totally, kind of needing Rhonda to make her feel good about herself. But, on the other hand, Rhonda's controlling ways and the things she said pissed her off majorly and Adult Naomi wanted to 'lock her off'*.

---

* '*Lock her off*' – to shut someone out of your life.

They also seemed to have the alcoholic-for-a-mum thing in common.

If you asked me, Rhonda's opinion mattered way too much and, from my point of view, she seemed to give Adult Naomi some serious headache if she didn't live up to her 'high expectations'.

The more I had read in the diaries about this 'best friendship', the more I began to realize that no one in Adult Naomi's life particularly liked Rhonda. In fact, some (family) disliked her immensely and felt she didn't have a positive influence on her life.

Still, I needed to know for myself and wanted to find out if Rhonda was really the Thelma to Adult Naomi's Louise.

Rhonda Simpson was curvy, with curly brown hair and hazel eyes. When she smiled, her face irradiated an unusual beauty. It made me want to smile too, which was a bit weird, considering I didn't know her, but I instantly relaxed, like I had with Danielle. This déjà vu was so strange, I decided to push it down as far as I possibly could.

Rhonda was happy to see me initially and then scolded me for her not being able to contact me over the past weeks. I lied and told her what I thought Adult Naomi might say, that I'd needed some time to get over French Dude. She wanted to know exactly what had happened between us, but not remembering, I mumbled something about it still being too painful, which she seemed to accept.

So instead, Rhonda spent pretty much most of the evening talking about her new boyfriend and I listened and nodded and tried to stop my mind from wandering. I knew she had one child and she was at her grandma's for the night, but again, she was a single mother and again, she pulled out the papers and a bag of weed and rolled a joint. I was just sitting there thinking, *What is it with all of these pothead friends?*

Her stories about this man bored me eventually; he didn't seem to be treating her well, but it was none of my business and I gave up trying to figure it or her out. It just made her sound self-absorbed and disinterested in Adult Naomi's life, and she seemed to hint that if it all went bad, it would some-how be Adult Naomi's fault. I *so* did not get this, but ignored her and tried to remember why I had visited in the first place. It took several attempts, but I managed to steer the conversa-tion round to the time before the '3Ds' diary. I asked her about her mum.

'Oh, she's fine, still the same.' She paused. 'Have you spoken to yours yet?'

'My mum?' I questioned. 'Oh no, not since . . .' I didn't know what to say.

'I know, so bad what she did, so naughty.'

'I know.' I tried not to look clueless. 'But you know . . .' I hesitated. 'I've just got to, you know, like, build a bridge and get over it.'

Rhonda looked shocked. 'Get over her telling you your dad isn't really your dad?'

I almost dropped the cup I was holding. 'What?' I splut-tered. Was she joking? 'What . . . what was she thinking, mad woman?' I tried to give a half-laugh and shake my head.

'Hmm.' She raised one eyebrow. 'Well, whatever she was thinking, to tell a lie like that is beyond forgivable.'

'Yeah,' I agreed. So frickin' Jekyll and Hyde offensive, bogus smeggin', majorly, majorly unforgivable. It was all starting to make sense. This was why she wasn't in Adult Naomi's life; it had to be. But why? Why would she say something like that?

I suddenly wanted to leave and to be with Leo and Simone, so I finished my drink, listened to Rhonda talk some more about her new boyfriend, called a taxi, and left. By the time I got back to Adult Naomi's house I decided I didn't want to phone and disturb Simone or Leo and could wait until I saw Simone to ask her some more about what had happened to Adult Naomi that summer.

Instead I lay in bed that night, thinking about her friends, what she had written about them in the diaries and how through her experiences they had ended up in her life. I thought about the car accident Maeve had spoken about and how upset Adult Naomi must have been, knowing she was going to lose her business. I thought of what Danielle said about 'Beautiful' dying and couldn't imagine what that must have been like, to be friends with someone you really respect and admire and eventually get close to them, only for them to be gone a year later. To top it all, having an alcoholic mother who had that many unresolved issues with Art that she felt the need to take it out on Adult Naomi. My dad wasn't my real dad! Was she for real?

I felt well sad and really sorry for Adult Naomi, and kinda sorry for her friends too. But it was obvious from being around them that Katie, Simone and Dean were her true friends. The others? Well, is that why she got so stoned around them? So that she could ignore the obvious fact that they had nothing in common?

They were really different from the friends I had back home

– *sooooo* different – and Adult Naomi really didn't fit in with them. I could see this from the diaries and the things she went through with them, but why couldn't she? It was all so confusing.

I closed my eyes and searched my mind for the familiar darkness of the house. It was still there, and the faint light still shone in the window. Finally, I could see the whole window, the bigger picture. Adult Naomi had given up on herself.

Why?

I turned towards the house.

The door was open.

8

Butterflies and Hurricanes

It's like you get stuck, you feel trapped and you can't see a way out,
and then a storm comes and beats you up,
knocks you back down.
But when it's gone and you're lying there beaten,
you realize you've become unstuck.
In all of the chaos
the storm has released you from the trap.

N. C.

I woke up feeling a mega sadness about everything I had read and heard so far.

Not just for Adult Naomi and the stuff she had been through that summer, but for her friends as well. What they had told me wasn't good and they all seemed to be struggling with some deep stuff of their own, with their only answer being to get high and put themselves in seriously smegged-up relationships. Was this happening to some women in the world? Were things that bad? Was this, like, because of the way the magazines were? Or this reality TV that *so* wasn't real life? It was all, like, one big personality contest, and whoever could humiliate the hardest and sex-tape the biggest and airbrush the best won the biggest prize. Everybody watching them.

I felt the opposite; I did want people to see me, but if they did, I didn't want to embellish or bandage – no, I wanted to stand at the top of the highest mountain and scream to everyone that would listen: *WAKE UP WORLD! THIS IS SO NOT RIGHT!*

Instead I did what I reckoned most people did. I retreated into my own world.

I spent hours and hours on the Internet watching videos uploaded by people from all over the world. Piano-playing cats, doped-up kids from the dentist, young girls using plastic cups as percussion instruments while singing, young boys with guitars, adults with their cars, women showing you how to 'get that look' with make-up. Teens skateboarding, snowboarding and sandboarding, looking for a sponsorship deal. Wannabe rappers and girls with voices like Mariah on talk shows looking for record deals.

What's the deal?

Then there were the UFO sightings, crop circles, conspiracy theories, secret societies, corrupt governments, radio shows, TV shows, Internet shows, podcasts, live feeds, realtime streaming . . . Downloads, uploads and loads and loads of . . . stuff!

Everybody had an opinion on something and there was a platform for that opinion. The Internet. It just seemed to me that everyone had, like, this desperate need to be heard; everyone was saying, *Look at me, can you hear me, can you see me? Am I here? Am I real? Do I matter?*

Andy Warhol was right: six and a half billion people were getting their fifteen minutes' of fame and okay, so, having aspirations to be a famous actress as a kid, I understood a little bit. But everyone's need to be famous had grown to a level I never would have imagined.

Was this what had happened to Adult Naomi? Was her need to be seen, to be heard, to be acknowledged so important to her that trying too hard had made her ill?

My only answer was to switch off the laptop and delve back into the diaries.

I picked up the one from 2005.

18 September 2005

I haven't written for a while, not since the night before the flashback. I can see the build-up to it and know what caused it. But I haven't told anyone about it and I'm not going to. This is all about boundaries; I always feel like my boundaries are walked all over. The argument with Simone, the argument with Karl, the argument with Eve. I constantly let people in and they always do something, they always cross a line, and I end up feeling like the little girl again, lost, lonely, abused and wondering what I have done so wrong to be attacked like that. Then in my fear of 'I need to protect myself from this, from you', I go ballistic and get confrontational and it all ends in tears.

It's like Leo's birthday all over again. The one time I ask for support from my friends and family, because Leo's dad upset me again, and what do they do? They get drunk in my home and start having raging arguments with each other. On my son's birthday! In my house! And then they

*blame each other, not taking responsibility for their actions.
And when I voice my disdain, I get laughed at, told to shut
up or told crap like your dad isn't your real dad.*

*I am so tired. I don't know who to trust. I'm crying
while writing this because I am so tired of it all. I wish my
body didn't hurt. I want the tension and the pain to stop
now. I don't want to go backwards anymore. No more
bad, dark, depressing suicidal places, no more boundary-
less territory, no more doing things for people in the name
of what I thought was love and now know isn't. What's
the point?*

*I'm losing the business – the accident has caused so
much pain. I am trying to keep it all together but the debt
is piling up.*

*And then to top it all, I have that god-almighty
flashback and well . . .*

I stopped reading and flicked through the pages before this
entry. Flashback? Flashback of what? What had happened?
There was nothing, no mention of it, just one small entry, the
beginnings of a letter.

13 August 2005

Dear Naomi,

*Little girl in the pink dress, I'm sorry that I've ignored
you. I'm sorry that I wanted you to stay hidden and away
from me and my life. I'm sorry that I have ignored your
pain and your need to heal. I understand the flashbacks
now, the one on the stairs yesterday and the one I had
today. Today it was a smell, a simple smell, but it took me*

*back to that flat where he lived and the way it used to
smell. Stale oil, musty but sickly sweet. It isn't quite
finished, is it? And I know now that if I deny you, you
will eventually push through and make me aware of the
boo boo. That eventually the boo boo needs healing and
I am the only one that can do it.*

What the hell is going on? I thought. *Flashbacks? Little girl
in the pink dress? Is this the 'inner child' I read about in the
other diaries? Is this me? What happened?*

I flicked through the pages again, searching for answers.
Nothing. Adult Naomi didn't write about it again. What came
after was the '3Ds' diary and then her leaving the house and
moving to Greece. I flicked the pages again and a piece of
paper dropped out of the middle of the diary. I hadn't noticed
it before. It was a typed letter, thin and worn like it had been
read over and over again.

It was from a mental health worker to a psychotherapist
and was about Adult Naomi.

Dear Catherine,

Thank you for your referral of this woman, who
presented with symptoms of low mood and low self-esteem
related to a history of abuse. I met her on three occasions
during October and November to make an initial
assessment, the outcome of which was to put her name
on our waiting list for individual psychotherapy.

Ms Jacobs is an intelligent and highly motivated woman,
who has many strengths and is functioning well in many
areas of her life. However, her self-esteem is very fragile, as

is her sense of 'self' in general, and at times of severe stress she has experienced a degree of fragmentation of her personality. This is particularly frightening for her because of a history of psychosis and mental illness in her family.

However, her difficulties can also be seen as a consequence of adverse early experiences which have damaged her self-esteem and affected her ability to manage internal distress. Hence Ms Jacobs can feel completely overwhelmed by powerful emotions, which can feel chaotic and frightening. She also experiences physical pain which seems to be connected to internal psychological states.

I am hopeful Ms Jacobs will be able to explore her difficulties within a safe therapeutic relationship with the aim of developing further her capacity to manage and contain distress without recourse to use cannabis, drugs or excessive painkillers. She is aware that therapy may increase her symptoms of anxiety and depression and that it will be important to discuss this with her therapist so that they, along with Ms Jacobs, can monitor the balance of risks–benefits of therapy. Ms Jacobs feels the risk of suicide is very low, as she is aware of the impact this would have on her son, and in recent months she has found adaptive ways of managing distress such as seeking help from her sister and/or the Samaritans.

Should you have any queries about my assessment or the proposed treatment, please do not hesitate to contact me.

With best wishes

Yours sincerely

Ms S. Libbert

I put the letter back into the diary and placed it on the shelf next to me.

Stopping my brain from even thinking about what I had just read, I got out of bed, ran a bath, climbed into it, washed my body, dried myself, and dressed in the *Miami Vice* velour tracksuit I'd turned my nose up at weeks ago. Then I went downstairs and had just made myself a cup of peppermint tea when the phone rang.

'Hiya, hun.' It was Simone.

'Hi,' I said quietly.

'What's up, Nay?' She knew instantly that something was wrong.

'Simone . . .' I took a deep breath and then burst into tears. 'What the hell happened to me?'

'What? What's wrong?'

It all came out in one big unpunctuated stream. 'The diaries the stories being depressed feeling suicidal being bipolar. I mean, what the . . . ? And the cocaine and smoking weed and Mum and her alcoholic lies and losing my home my business. Why? And then the friends and the arguments and the flashbacks.' I sobbed. 'Low self-esteem no sense of self what the hell is fragmentation of personality and abuse? Abuse? What abuse?'

'Nay.'

'And then psychotherapy and needing help and not having anyone to help me and . . . STRESS! BLOODY STRESS AGAIN!'

'Nay—'

'And the flashbacks? Flashbacks to what?'

'Nay, listen to me—'

'Flashbacks to what?' I bawled.

'NAOMI JACOBS!' Simone shouted this time.

I stopped talking but the tears carried on, silently.

'Listen, babe, just take a deep breath and calm down. Nay, breathe.'

I did and exhaled into a quiet sob.

'Listen, hun, I'm coming up in about an hour. I was calling to say I'll go shopping, cook a Sunday roast for us all and I'll stay over.' She spoke softly.

'Okay,' I whispered.

'Nay, this is all the past. It's history, remember. I know it's not to you. I know it feels like the future, but it's not. This has already happened and you're reading about it, but it doesn't have to affect you *now* in a bad way, okay?'

'Okay.' I didn't understand. I *was* affected by what I had read, affected in a big way.

'What I mean is, babe, it's your choice. It's your choice how you deal with this. If it's too much, stop. It's that simple; put down the diaries and stop reading. You've done a lot this weekend; give yourself a break. You don't need to know everything right now, okay?'

I thought about what Katie had said, about hospital, but after what I had just read, I had images of men in white coats, large needles, and padded rooms.

No way, Jose. Leo. I had a child to take care of. I needed to pull it together.

'No, I'm okay.'

'Are you sure?' she asked.

'Yeah, you're right; it's just all a bit overwhelming. I'm gonna step away from the diaries.' I faked a laugh. 'Is Leo okay?'

'Oh, he's great, Nay. We've had a laugh today. He's been making papier mâché masks with his mates. He's made one for you.'

Thoughts of Leo being happy quelled the flow of tears.

'Nay, please remember that no matter what has happened, you have done a bloody fantastic job with him. You should be so proud, 'cause you've raised a beautiful, smart and funny boy, and he's a credit to you, do you hear me?'

'Y . . . Y . . . Yes,' I stuttered.

'No, I mean it. Don't you ever forget that,' she insisted.

'Okay, thanks, Sim.'

'Right, we'll be up in a bit, and give the diaries a rest, okay?'

'Okay.'

'Love you.'

'I love you too.'

And I meant it. I felt right there and then that despite what I had read in the diaries about the arguments we had had over the years and the not speaking for months, that when the universe was handing out sisters, I had been at the front of the queue and had struck gold. But true to form, I ignored her pleas to put the diaries down and went straight back upstairs. I had a feeling I was close to understanding why I was here.

It took me an hour and a half to flick through the other diaries and search through the boxes of letters and printed emails Adult Naomi had stashed under her bed. I was gathering the centre-pieces of the puzzle. A picture was beginning to form. And then I found some pieces of paper; they were pages ripped out of her 2002 diary.

8 April 2002

I've been told that if I write it down, how it's affected my life, then maybe it will somehow help. So here goes.

I am still affected by it in many ways; the fact that I can't remember exactly what happened pains me. It comes in dribs and drabs. A memory here, a flashback there. It makes me feel stupid at times and leads me to seriously doubt myself. I know I have a low sense of self-worth. I find it hard to maintain my self-esteem and confidence. It never feels real. Like it's mine. It's like it doesn't belong to me.

I still have feelings of dirtiness; I have since I was a child, like no matter what I do I could never get clean. It's not as bad as it used to be, though. Maybe it's getting better the more I remember.

I go through periods of hating myself with a passion, and although most times I don't even realize it, I have a low opinion of myself. I do not believe I deserve success or can achieve my goals. My depression isn't that bad right now, but I still smoke weed when I panic and feel out of control of the things in my life. I think my life is blessed, but I cut off when I do something good; when people praise me I do not believe them, that it's really me doing it. I am not able to enjoy feeling good and find it hard to trust my intuition, to trust myself and others. I constantly strive for perfection but often don't finish the things I start, which makes me feel like a failure. My feelings scare me sometimes because I don't understand them. I don't understand where they come from. I feel very attached and then very detached. I can think violent thoughts and

*get so angry with myself. I have felt suicidal many times;
even now I still get very confused at times and panic
about making decisions.*

I turned over the page.

*My mum is an alcoholic and I buy her drink when she
visits. I know I do this for her approval, so that I feel like
she'll love me just a little bit more. So that she can see I
understand her.*

*My sister still lives with me, and I know we need to
come apart because we rely on each other too much but
I don't want her to leave. What would happen to me if
she did? What would happen to Leo? Am I enough of a
mother and father for him?*

*I feel very cut off from people and the world at times.
I go out and dance because I need to feel something, feel
that I'm sexy, because I have never been happy with my
body or the way it looks. I feel like my body has betrayed
me, it has let me down.*

*I still think I am a bad person and I don't deserve the
love I am shown. I get anxious and tense if a person sits
too close to me, touches me, etc. I usually at some point
before, during or after sex quietly panic and hold my
breath.*

*I smoke weed when I am sad or in pain and have
always had this unexplainable pain in my body that I
know comes from my mind. Because it starts, always
starts, with a thought. I think this is in some way
connected to the abuse. None of my relationships last*

*long and I don't think I make any real friends because
I don't share who I am with people.*

I found another ripped page.

*I sleep sometimes when I am coping. I know I am coping
because I sleep; dreaming helps me to cope. But it doesn't
happen very often. I don't think I have had a proper
night's sleep for twenty years.*

   *I try and cope by immersing myself in my son's world,
becoming a child again, playing with him, wrestling,
tickling him, making him laugh, reading stories to him,
painting, building things with him, watching his favourite
films with him. Making up stories where he is always the
hero – he loves this. We play football together, even in
the rain; we put our wellies on and go out and splash
in the puddles and play Pooh sticks.*

   We bake cakes and then eat them until we are stuffed.

   *I cope by giving myself the childhood I wanted. By
being the mother I always needed.*

The way Adult Naomi felt about herself majorly wigged me
out for a moment there; so much negative stuff. But in a weird
way, I kind of got it. If she was in pain, I understood why she
didn't feel good about herself. It also began to explain why
three years later, in 2005, she began to lose it. I mean, having
to deal with everybody else's crap as well as feeling like she
did. No wonder she couldn't cope. I still didn't get the drugs
thing, but if she didn't rate herself highly, then maybe that's
all she felt like she deserved in her life. If you can't *feel* good,

how do you *know* what good is? Still, she found ways to cope sometimes, which was a good thing, right?

But what happened to her? I turned the page. And what I read flipped everything in my fifteen-year-old world upside down.

> *You . . .*
>
> *You abused my trust and stole my innocence. You stole a part of me which I now struggle to get back every day of my life. I hate you. I hate the abuse I now inflict on myself because of you. I am alone and I have to deal with this on my own and I'm scared. Scared of going to bed early, scared of being on my own, scared of other people's thoughts of me, scared of myself. I have buried all of this pain for far too long. It feels like it's fucked me up in ways I can't describe and I feel like you have won. Sometimes I get one over on you, sometimes I feel like I am winning and I can never go back to that place you put me, but then I find myself there and realize you've won again. I hate you. I don't care who hurt you or abused you. You had no right to do it to me; you had no right to touch me in places that belonged to me. Why did you rape me? I didn't do anything wrong to you. All of that hate and anger pushed onto me, forced into me, and then you told me not to cry. That it was my fault, that I was a dirty little bitch. HOW DARE YOU!*
>
> *There's no health here; there's no health in my mind, in my body, in my heart. You took my health and I want it back, it's not yours; it wasn't yours to take and yet something made you think it was. I blamed myself;*

*I thought it was me, that I did it all. But I know now
it wasn't. It was you.*

   It was you . . .
   You!
   NO . . . no . . . no . . . no . . . no

I searched through the box again; this couldn't be true.
Stole my innocence?
NO.
What happened to her?
. . . touch me in places that belonged to me.
NO!
Not her, not me, not this!
. . . forced into me, and then you told me not to cry.
NO!
I picked up the box and threw it against the wall. The rest
of the papers flew out.

NO! I slumped against the wall and let out a loud scream.
'NO!'

The only words going around my head: *It wasn't yours to
take.*

A cold darkness seemed to cover my body and wrap its icy
hands around me. I couldn't breathe. I grabbed at my chest,
gasping for air. Sobs caught in my throat and I desperately
tried to push them out, but my body seemed to be fighting the
pain, wanting to push it down, push it further inside.

I lay on the floor amongst the papers and diaries and curled
into a ball. It reminded me of all those weeks ago when I first
woke up in the future and had lain on the bathroom floor
thinking I was stuck, trapped like a caterpillar in the chrysalis

of an intricately spun nightmare. Caught in a bad, wicked, terrible dream that I had no control over. This was ten times worse.

I cried until I had no choice but to give in to the pain; it found its way out. All of the fear, frustration and furiousness flooded out of me, drowning me, drowning the mental images of the diary pages, into one bottomless pit of waste matter.

Is this why I am here? Is this what I woke up in the future to find out, that I was abused as a child?

NO! It can't be; this can't be happening. Adult Naomi . . .

I needed Adult Naomi.

I sat up, my face soaked with tears, my body drenched in sweat, and picked up my hand to wipe my face. A page was stuck to it. It was then that I saw three more pages sticking out from under the bed. It had Adult Naomi's writing on it. Feeling too weak to sit upright, I leaned against the wall and read the papers.

16 September 2005

I'm sat in the car outside the school waiting for Callie to get here with the keys. It's raining. I'm early, the first one here. I felt like writing, but I don't have my journal, so am using the back of one of my worksheets to write this. Have been sat here thinking about everything I have been through this summer. The therapy with Ben, he teaching me to see my mind as a house, to help me find the hidden parts. The parts I buried so deep, so long ago. He did say it may get worse before it gets better. Boy, I didn't realize how much worse it could get. Although once you open Pandora's Box, it's near impossible to close it. But when

Leo was born I made a promise to myself that I would heal whatever pain was inside of me, that I would give him a better life than I've had. To heal whatever wounds needed healing, no matter how bad they were. It took me four years to pluck up the courage but I did it. It's the reason why I started this therapy: to remember.

I wanted to know. I needed to know. And well, now I do. The flashback last month on the stairs confirmed it. It makes sense now, why I have never liked wearing pink. I was wearing a pink dress when the sexual assault happened.

I've been thinking about trust while sat here. About how trusting children are, how trusting I was. He wasn't a family member or even a friend. But he was the brother of a friend and he was trusted. Was it because he was married and a member of the church? Didn't anybody suspect him? Those days were different then; parents never suspected if they left their children with people that they would come to harm, and certainly not sexual. But I did; he harmed me, assaulted me, and I saw how deeply and painfully he did during that flashback. So painfully that I saw my mind actually splitting when he raped me all those years ago and the sheer force of that memory made me fall down the stairs, and by the time I reached the bottom I was six years old again. How does that happen? I left my body, my adult body, and six-year-old me came back from the past and had full control. I could see what was happening to me as I floated above. But I couldn't get back into my body.

I haven't told anyone, not even Ben. I just don't

understand how this could happen to me, how I could leave my body like that. I am just grateful it didn't last that long, and that it was the photo of Leo on the wall that pulled me back into my body, brought the adult me back into the present. But now she's here, the little girl in the pink dress, six-year-old me, with me, inside of me, inside the house; she calls it the 'boo boo' what he did to her, to me, and she needs healing. I need healing. Maybe this is why my relationship with Eve and her drinking has always felt so chaotic and abusive, because of what I went through as a small child. How did I survive it? I was only six. But I get it now, it just makes sense; I get why I've always hated the colour pink – I associate it with vulnerability. I understand the drugs, the weed-smoking, the depression. The flashback was horrible – it was like going through it all over again – but if I hadn't have had it, well, I wouldn't understand right now. So much is starting to make sense.

I also remembered something the other day when I was with Callie; we were talking about when we were kids and our favourite books. I was thinking about Jonathan Livingston Seagull *and how profoundly it had affected me, and then I thought about how it kind of saved me really. I remember being ten years of age and trusting again, and again that trust being violated twice by another 'friend' of the family. Someone completely different but someone who again thought they had the right to abuse my trust and cross the adult–child boundary. The shame and disgust I felt when he kissed me, forcing his tongue into my mouth, made me turn inwards and to books and to food. But it was that book that told me there was something in life to look forward to. That one day I would get away and live my life, really live, soaring high above like Jonathan, and I would be free. Am I free now? Has remembering all of this freed me? I don't feel free. There's too much pain to feel free. Maybe one day I will.*

Maybe.

I feel like crying right now, but I can't, I have a class to teach. I need to get it together. You know, if I think about it, I really didn't stand a chance; these were my experiences before I even knew about boys, and eventually when I did meet a boy he ended up trying to kill me – my first boyfriend tried to strangle the life out of me, while he was under the influence of drugs. I often wonder what would have happened if his best friend hadn't pulled him off me.

Well, I wouldn't be here writing this.

And through all of this, the only thing I ever wanted was for my dad to come and get me, and take me away from these bad men. Except that never happened, so instead I buried it.

Ben says that maybe I seek men out who remind me of my dad because I feel I need rescuing, that the little girl inside me still needs rescuing. And I do, you know. Even Karl, the break-ups and then the make-ups and the arguments . . . we seem to be going around in the same circle. I am the victim, he is my rescuer, and then everything is okay for a while. Until it begins again. But my dad is the only man I have ever trusted, the only man I feel safe around. I don't know what to do.

And, well, the worst of it came out on the stairs last month. That was different, that was a flashback on a whole other level. A level I don't understand. Why did my mind split like that?

Maybe I need to tell someone. I might tell Georgie – she's my fellow psychology student; maybe she can figure out what it was. I think maybe this is the real reason I am studying psychology, so that eventually I can stop depending on therapy and become my own therapist.

Maybe.

Callie's just pulled up in her car. Well, uni starts next month. I will talk to Georgie then, fresh start. I have a good job, a business that is going well, a beautiful son, and a great boyfriend. Maybe things will only get better from here on out.

Yeah, they can only get better.

Maybe.

But they didn't.

I put the paper down; the grey afternoon clouds outside made the room feel dark. It felt empty, devoid of life, numb, like me. The tears had stopped. I wiped my face and tried to think, but my mind was blank. I didn't know what to do and I didn't know where to go.

Outside, I heard the faint sound of Simone's car door close and Leo calling the cat to him. After splashing my face with cold water, I rushed down the stairs to see Leo taking off his shoes at the door.

'Hiya, Leo,' I said, hoping he wouldn't notice my swollen eyes. He looked up at me and the smile on his face immediately wiped any sad thoughts from my mind. He was so happy to see me.

'Oooh, I've missed you.' I threw my arms around him and squeezed him tight.

'I made you a mask.' He pulled it out from behind his back. Colourfully and carefully decorated in green and blue with glitter and feathers on, it looked like something I would wear to a Mardi Gras.

'Wow.' I looked at it in awe and then at him. 'You did this? No way, Jose.'

He nodded proudly. 'Yeah, I made one for me as well, but mine's more of a boy's one. Look, it's got the Brazil colours on it.' He took a yellow-, blue- and green-painted one from his bag and handed it to me.

'Oh my dayz! Leo Jacobs, you are, like, *sooooo* talented; you're, like, this mega awesome artist. Who knew? Have you been keeping secrets from me?' I asked him.

He giggled and shook his head. We walked into the living room together. Simone was already in the kitchen, putting the shopping away.

'Yeah, you know I'm good at art, Mum, like Granddad and JJ and Simone,' he said matter-of-factly.

'I know, but these are on, like, another level, so wicked.' I stared at the masks, beaming.

'And we went skateboarding and I did a kickflip one-eighty,' he stated proudly.

'Shut the front door! Really?' I had no clue what he was talking about. 'What did your mates think?'

'Oh, they know I'm good at boarding, no biggy. I'm gonna try a heelflip next time.' He laughed and went into the kitchen.

'Kriss biscuits. Nice one, top one.' I followed him in awe,

thinking, *Where does this kid get his confidence from?* I watched him make himself a juice, while Simone told me of their weekend.

Leo placed his glass by the sink.

'Can I go and play on my Xbox, Mum?' He widened his eyes, reminding me of a cute puppy dog.

'Err . . .' My instinct was to look at Simone, but I really wanted to be his mum at that moment and make this small but significant decision. 'Have you got any homework?' Yes, that's what mums would say.

He looked up at the ceiling and retrieved the answer from his ten-year-old memory bank. 'Naaa, did it all on Friday.'

'Cool; go on then,' I said.

'Yes!' He was out of the kitchen and upstairs faster than Linford Christie.

'You all right, sis?' Simone walked over to me and gave me a big hug.

I sank into her arms and gave a deep sigh. 'Yeah, I am now that you guys are here.'

She pulled back and took a good look at me and, in true Simone style, like a bartender doling out advice to a drunk customer, she gave it to me straight, no chaser. 'You look awful.'

I laughed. 'That's what will happen to you when you cry loads while reading that half of your life has been really smegged up and most of it is full of tosser crap that's sent your mind bipolar-bear mental.'

Simone laughed. 'Bipolar bear?'

'Well, I've gotta laugh, sis. If I don't, well, I think it will send me like . . . like Loopy Larry.'

'Loopy Larry?'

'*Do you have a penny, missus?*' I reminded her and held out my hand.

'Oh my God, I'd forgotten about him,' she chuckled. 'Nay, things won't ever get that bad.'

'They nearly did. I mean, look at me now; she's totally left the building and I'm like fifteen AGAIN! Like the first time she left wasn't bad enough, Adult Naomi has some frickin' need to split and leave me here.'

'What do you mean?'

I knew I was talking about the adult me in the third person again, but Simone didn't seem disturbed by it.

'Well, this has happened before.' My throat was tightening; my eyes were beginning to burn.

'Before?' Simone frowned, and from her face, I could tell she had no clue. 'When?'

'Three years ago, 2005, except it only lasted for an hour and she was six again, and she didn't tell anyone until she told Georgie at uni, and then Georgie suggested she go and see someone, like a psychiatrist.'

'Oh, right, okay.' Simone went quiet. This was the first time she was hearing of this, I could tell.

'And then, like, well, all that stuff about when I was little . . . I don't remember.' The tears fell. 'Someone hurt her, Sim. Hurt me, like really hurt me.'

She stepped to me and held me tightly while I cried. 'I know, babe, I know.'

'And I don't know what to do now. I mean, why am I fifteen again? Is it because of what happened? Do I have to do something? I don't understand what's happening.'

'What did Adult Naomi do?' If this third person concept was strange to her, she seemed to accept it.

'What do you mean?' I released myself from my sister's embrace and sought the kitchen paper. 'Total snot fest,' I said, mocking my dripping nose.

'Look, you're still laughing, even though you're feeling . . .'

'Majorly sad.' I blew my nose.

'Yeah.' Simone smiled. 'So what would you – I mean, Adult Naomi – do?'

I thought about it for a second and what I'd read about her in the diary entries. 'Get frickin' high most probably,' I said bitterly.

'Yeah, but that's not an option.'

'Oh, hell no,' I agreed. The way I felt, I would never pick up another spliff as long as I lived.

I thought for a while longer. Her friends were out of the picture for now. Katie had four children to deal with. Dean was away on his music travels. Eve was gone and had no clue what was happening and hadn't for the past four years. Art was a motorway ride away and had no clue what was going on. I didn't want to read a book or watch a DVD.

There was a loud crash and a bang from the floor above us. Leo. Of course, duh!

I looked at Simone as if I had just been searching for my glasses and found them on my head.

I went to the bottom of the stairs. 'Are you okay, son?' I shouted up. It was the first time I had called him 'son' and I liked it.

'Yeah,' he shouted back. 'It was my Xbox games; they fell off my shelf.'

'Oh, okay.'

I looked up at the photos on the wall and that was when I had my own first memory. I didn't know whether it was because of what I had read in the diary pages, if it was a flashback, or some weird flashforward, but it was like a screen had flipped down and someone was projecting an image onto a white canvas. I could see Adult Naomi clearly lying at the bottom of the stairs. It wasn't this house; it was another house. The carpet colour was different. She was half naked because she had just got out of the bath, and was wrapped in a towel and had fallen down the stairs. She was distressed, scared, and in pain and, yes, in her mind, she was six years old again and didn't know where she was or what to do. Adult Naomi was, like, there, but not – the part of her mind that was her was watching from above, cut off from her body. She had no control over what was happening. The six-year-old girl had control and lay there for ages, scared and confused. Then she saw a photograph of Leo on the wall above her and it brought her back into the moment. It made her realize she was in the future and she needed to let go and let Adult Naomi back into her body.

Seeing this made me feel dizzy, so I sat on the bottom step of the stairs, realizing that this *had* happened before. It hadn't happened to me. But it had happened to Adult Naomi. It had happened to this body I was in.

It made me think of the letter: *fragmentation of her personality.*

So it was a picture of Leo that saved her, stopped it from happening. Until now.

I stared at Leo's wellington boots.

'Leo,' I shouted up to him.

'Yes, Mum?'

Mum. Cool! 'Do you wanna go to the park with me?'

'The park?' He came to the top of the stairs. 'It's raining.'

'I know, but we've got boots.'

He shook his head 'Naaa.'

I felt despondent.

'Actually . . .' He came back to the top of the stairs. 'Let me finish this level and we'll go.'

'Safe.' I jumped up and pulled my Ugly boots on.

Leo and I went to the park under the clouds of a soft drizzle rain and splashed in the puddles. We played in the mud, making shapes with twigs, and tried to guess each other's pictures. We fed stale bread to the ducks and geese by the lake and nuts to the squirrels. The swings and roundabouts were wet and slippery, but it didn't stop us from jumping on them and laughing loudly, while the spinning motion made our stomachs flip over. We told each other jokes. He didn't get mine, and I laughed at his anyway.

The sun came out eventually and three rainbows formed. I told Leo of how I had once followed a rainbow and actually found an end. It had lit up the grass and the trees and everywhere had a golden glow and I had felt magical, special even, that I had found the end of a rainbow. Leo reminded me of the time Adult Naomi had found a four-leaf clover before she started her holistic therapy business and Art had framed it for her. I pretended to remember and stated that I was lucky in my life, especially lucky to have a child like him.

He smiled and went off to make mud castles while I swung on the swings and watched him. Adult Naomi had been through so much in her life, so much crap. But I reckoned that Leo made it all right, that whatever she couldn't do for herself, she did for Leo, and I knew deep down that she had made sure he'd got the life she never had. I was glad she'd stuck it out and that she had somehow protected him from a lot of what she had been through. She was a good mum, it was obvious, but I think somewhere along the way, Adult Naomi had forgotten herself. She had forgotten who she really was. But, I thought, had she ever really known?

We arrived home a couple of hours later, wet, muddy, but happy. I felt so much better, lighter and free. Simone, Leo and I ate a lovely roast dinner, watched a movie, and played Monopoly. We laughed all night and then I put Leo to bed.

'Tell me another story, Mum.' Leo pulled the covers up to his chin.

I sat on the edge of his bed and thought for a while, and then I told him a story of a brother and sister, who were a skateboarding-loving prince and a hip-hop music-loving princess, but the princess was kidnapped by a wicked witch and given a forgetting potion. She forgot who she was and lived as a house servant for the witch and had to cook lots and lots of pigeons because that was all the witch would eat. Everyone thought she was dead, but the brother never gave up looking for her and eventually, while disguised as a market seller who sold wood for skateboards, he found her. But she didn't remember him and didn't trust him. The brother had to slay a big bad scary dragon to get the dragon's tooth, which could be made into a potion to help his sister remember. He did and then used the dragon scales as armour to protect him when the witch tried to stop him. The brother and sister both killed the witch and he gave the potion to his sister. She remembered him and they went back home to the kingdom where everyone was happy and celebrated the return of the princess. Of course, the kingdom had massive skateboard ramps, and Snoop Doggy Dogg and Dr Dre came especially to perform for the princess.

Leo thought my story was fantastic and it reminded me of when I was little and used to tell my sister stories to help her fall asleep. I always felt good when I did. Telling stories had always helped me.

That night, I sat in a hot bath and looked down at the body I had woken up in. Adult Naomi's body, my body. I was tired and sad, but now I understood everything. Adult Naomi was sexually abused and assaulted when she was six years of age and it was the first time her mind had split from her body. This body.

It happened again when she was ten. That was why she had turned to books and food.

Is this why I binged then threw up all the time?

She had a boyfriend who tried to kill her?

Tried to strangle the air from this body.

I put my hand to my neck and I understood why, by the time she was eighteen, she had turned to drugs.

The heat from the water felt good. I took a deep breath in and watched my abdomen fill with air; I breathed out and watched it lay flat. The water massaged over it.

This body has been abused with drugs; she buried it all under drugs.

And then Leo was born.

This body had carried a baby, a big baby, and gave birth. I looked at my breasts. They had fed the baby, nurtured and comforted him.

This body was a mum, is a mum.

Leo.

He was the reason she had counselling, so she could be better for him, could make sure he got the life she never had. I held my breath and pulled my head under. The water separated my hair. She had counselling; she needed to know, she needed to understand her mind. She needed to find a way to heal it.

My head relaxed and I shook it from side to side. The water felt like fingers massaging my scalp. I understood why she was doing the psychology degree. It wasn't because she wanted to be a psychologist; it was so that she could understand the mind, her mind.

This body was hurt, damaged, and the pressure from all the buried pain caused the 'fragmentation of her personality' when, for an hour, she was six years old again. It was what she was afraid of and couldn't talk about in her diary. My lungs felt as if they were going to burst. I pulled my face out of the water and took a deep breath in.

I thought about the psychologists, the psychiatrists, the psychotherapists that had tried to help this body and mind, but in the end, hadn't really helped.

They said it was bipolar disorder.

I placed my palms on my face and closed my eyes. I tried to see inside my body. It hadn't slept properly in years – days and nights of no sleep, and then nights and days of nightmare-filled dreams. It hadn't eaten properly for years – constant diet changes, throwing up, not eating for days, meat one day, vegan the next.

But it's still here. It's still intact.

I moved my hands from my face to the handles on the side of the bath and pulled myself up. The water trickled down my body back into the bath.

Adult Naomi had tried – she had tried to save this body, and she had tried to save her mind. Moving to a new country to start again had been her only option, but it didn't work and she had to come back.

And that's when I think she gave up on herself.

I got out of the bath and towel-dried my body, silently thanking it for still being here, still surviving. I got into my PJs and lay on the bed, thinking about everything that had happened on the weekend: meeting Adult Naomi's friends, experiencing the future world again, and trying to understand her mind through the diaries. Before I closed my eyes and drifted off, I picked up the same diary that had the ripped pages missing from it. The 2002 diary.

9 April 2002

Dear Naomi,

 I want to heal you and mother you and make you feel better, and I know I will. I am trying. Please be patient with me and give me time; this is gonna take time, but it will happen, we will get through this. The universe is on our side; the divine spirit, the healing energies that exist will continue to come to us. I know that you are still hurt and angry and upset and in pain. I know that you are still in denial about some parts, but the healing will continue, the anger will cease and one day you will learn to love you. The abuse will stop. You will learn to listen to what you want, and how to listen to what you need. I can do that for you. It's not hard; I do it for Leo every day, for my loved ones. If I can do it for them, then I can do it for you.

I promise I will learn.

I promise.

> *Love always,*
> *Naomi x*

As I slipped into sleep, I realized that my questions had been answered. I knew as much about Adult Naomi as I needed to know and understood her as much as I ever would. I understood why she had made the decisions she had made, why she had surrounded herself with those so-called friends, and I now knew about her painful wounds inflicted by others that she had struggled to make better, to heal. I no longer felt sorry for her; I just felt major respect for what she had been through and the fact that she had survived it. I didn't need to know any more.

I had gained access to the house.

I found myself wandering in the darkness, through the hallways, searching for the light, asking one last question.

Why fifteen?

9
Looking Through the Darkness

Sometimes it's scary,
sometimes it's a fight,
but you've got to feel
through the darkness
to find the light.

L. C.

I woke up still thinking, why fifteen? Why was I now in the future at fifteen? I mean, it's not an age to swing your pants about.

At first, before I wanted to be a journalist, I wanted to be an actress. I was a bit of a drama queen, yeah, but I also thought I'd be a good actress because I was a bundle of nerves when I was a kid. I used to do this strange thing every time I would get tense: I'd smile, but more like bare my teeth, so what better profession to go into than acting?

I was thinking this while I ironed Leo's uniform the next morning and made him a sausage sandwich, remembering all that had happened to me from the age of ten. I walked with

Leo to school and thought about my school and how it was a safe haven for me, how much I loved being there. And how much I loved going to my friends' posh houses and feeling safe under their roofs with their 'normal' parents.

When I first woke up in the future Simone told me about Adult Naomi's small two-bedroom council house being a place of safety, a sanctuary for her. Even though it wasn't the house I thought I'd be living in by the time I was thirty-two, it was beginning to have the same effect on me. I felt safe when I was in this house. Was this the same for Adult Naomi's mind? Was this the reason I kept seeing the house, because she had felt the need to create a sanctuary for her mind, to give it a place to escape to?

As I turned the key in the door, I thought about Adult Naomi's diaries. I so got why she carried on writing. So much was going on inside of her head and if she couldn't speak her mind to people, she needed to get it out somehow. And then I had this thought that maybe if I carried on writing in them, then it might help me. It might even be what Adult Naomi needed to come back.

I found her 2008 diary in the drawer of the small table next to her bed. I sat on her bed and opened the diary to the next blank page. As soon as I started to write I began to remember what some of my life was like, and the words just quickly spilled out of me, like they were waiting to be written.

15 June 2008

Dear Adult Naomi,

If one day you read this, I want to let you know that I get it. I understand why you left. I hope one day you come back, but in case you don't, I think I should carry on the diaries for you, and because I think it will help me. If I remember stuff about me, then maybe I will know why I am here, you know? Anyway, I thought I would write what I can remember, which isn't much; it seems my head has been filled with your stuff the past couple of months. Today I started to think about mine, so here goes . . .

Last year . . . well, no, the year before . . . well, when I was thirteen, I kinda stopped hiding behind books. Remember I had that party, in the big hall, and I wore that hat and red lipstick and I thought I looked like Janet Jackson? I felt well kriss! It made me more popular at school; people wanted to know me and invite me to their parties. I felt free, you know, when I was around them, my friends, in their big posh houses. I could be myself. And then remember drama club, me acting? Playing someone else always felt better than being me. I could be whoever I wanted to be.

And then when I was fourteen everything changed. Do you remember the summer of the musical when I ended up on the front page of the local newspaper and singing on a kids' television show? The show was filmed in Manchester! No way, Jose! And you ended up coming to live here! I was also chosen for the grand finale and sang the closing number in the musical. I loved that summer – my time to shine. I felt well confident, had kind of a big head, but it was all frickin' fantastic.

It made me well sad to read that things didn't get

better with Mum, but last year I offered her out*,
remember? I'd had enough of the beatings I'd received
over the years; belt, slipper, umbrella, you name it, if it
was in the vicinity when we were in the throes of an
argument, she would reach for it and go ballistic. Oh, and
the constant blaming me for everything that Joseph's kids
or Simone did wrong . . . well, I just had to stick up for
myself more. It just felt so bloody unfair, you know. And
then there was that time I told her I was sick of her
smeggin' hitting me and to get outside where we would
fight one on one with fists only. I was crapping myself but
she walked away mortified and didn't hit me again. Well
sad, but I kinda understand why things turned out the
way they did.

But then things went a bit mental, didn't they?
Remember when I applied to a stage school in London
and they wrote to me saying my application was
successful and would I come down to London to do an
audition? Mum said no full stop.

Wasn't gonna be a famous actress then, so I kinda
went off the rails and started to argue with the teachers.
I wore more make-up (God, remember the way Mrs
O'Shea used to go on at me about my red lipstick? Didn't
she call me a harlot?) and I accidently on purpose spilt
bleach on my gross nun's skirt so I could buy a shorter
one.

Remember totally fit Robert Harris? And the rest of the
crew? And then the boys that liked me from that estate

---

* To 'offer someone out' – a Scouse term for challenging someone to a fist fight.

*me and Lydia used to hang out on? Well, I didn't wanna
be rescued then, I just wanted to snog boys! And then I
started to lie to Eve about where I was, so that I could
stay out late on a weekend.*

   *In the end I was skiving off school ALL the time.
Remember I didn't turn up for a month near the end of
fourth-year seniors, until one day I went in out of
boredom and Mr Frye, the head of year, sat me down and
told me that if I didn't buckle down and actually attend
school, I was gonna fail all of my GCSEs?*

   *I don't know why but it worked, didn't it? I started to
make an effort to study hard, catch up and pass my
exams. It was gonna be a cinch, I was gonna sail through
the exams. I was on the right track for all As by the end of
the fifth year and sack it, if I couldn't be an actress, I was
gonna be a journalist and travel the world reporting on
people and places.*

   So what happened?

   What happened to me? I wish I could remember.

      Love,

         Teen Nay x

There were still more diaries to look at, and one in particular that I wanted to read – a red diary. I knew instantly when
I found it at the bottom of the box that it was from 1991 and
1992. This was the diary *I'd* written in and the only one left
in the collection that I hadn't read yet. But I stuck to Simone's
advice that I should take a break and instead concentrated on
writing my own entries in the 2008 diary instead.

   During the days I immersed myself in Leo's world, walking

him to school, watching him skateboard, playing Xbox games with him and sometimes taking him to the park where we would swing on the swings and tell each other stories.

I even went to the massive Tesco and tried to get my head around all of the choice. Leo pretty much liked the same things as me so it was easy to shop for him and as I still couldn't figure out what my stomach wanted, I stuck to soups and sandwiches and jacket potatoes. These were the only things stopping me from hurling all over the place.

A letter came one morning reminding Adult Naomi of the psychology exams she was supposed to take, but there was no way I was gonna be able to do them. I thought telling the uni people that she had disappeared from her own mind and I had taken her place might have sounded a bit too tapped so I put it away.

I avoided most of Adult Naomi's friends because I *sooooo* didn't wanna talk to them. Not in a bad way; I just didn't know what to say to them. And I thought if I didn't smoke a spliff at some point, they would suspect something. If any of them called for something and they couldn't get through, they called Simone anyway and she dealt with them.

Katie and I spent some evenings talking about all the things I had read in the diaries. She knew more than I thought and filled in a lot of the blanks for me. But she confirmed that everything the diaries told me had happened to Adult Naomi was real and that she had been through a lot of it on her own. It still made me well sad, but almost, like, in awe of her as well, that she'd survived all of that crap and was still here. Well, technically, but not mentally. Still, I had to give the woman serious props!

Like with Dean, Katie and I somehow found the funny side of it all and I laughed like a moron into my herbal tea. If I didn't laugh, I would have cried, and I was so over crying.

Simone came and stayed and we had a lazy weekend watching Adult Naomi's *Buffy the Vampire Slayer* box sets. During the episode where Buffy's mum dies, Simone's mobile phone rang.

It was Nat and Marcy, our long-lost cousins. They had found each other at first through a lost family website and had got in touch with Simone a few months before, but Simone hadn't told me about them because she didn't want to cause any more stress or put pressure on me to remember, given the state of my brain. They had both been born to my mum's younger sisters and adopted out as babies and were searching for the family they never knew.

When Simone told me about them I wanted to talk to them, so called them the next day. It was really nice to speak to them both. When I was little I used to think about one day seeing my cousin Nat again. I didn't remember her, but in a weird way remembered loving her, and I kept a picture of her, part of a photo that was taken of us when we were babies and her Mum had lived with us in Liverpool for a while. It was an old picture split into four and I found out after all these years that she had kept the part of the photo with me in it. The bond had never been broken, and another cousin, Marcy, appearing was an added bonus.

I chatted to both of them for about an hour. They explained that some of the family spazzed out majorly when they turned up looking for them, but I was made up that they had found us. Eve's side of the family were so fractured and distant.

Living in different parts of the country and not seeing or talking to each other for years meant that the younger ones hadn't really grown up with the older ones, so they weren't close.

There were seven sisters; Evelyn was the eldest, then Paula, Gina, Annette, Rebecca, Meryl and Betty. United, they were a force to be reckoned with, a force that could rip a village apart and lay waste to everything. But divided, if they had a falling out, well, no one wanted to get in the middle because they knew it wasn't worth their lives. I called them 'The Sisters', although I only really knew two of my mum's sisters: Aunty Gina and Aunty Rebecca, who still lived in Liverpool and would sometimes visit us in the summer.

The story I used to hear being whispered was that 'The Sisters' were young girls when their African father died and they were all taken into foster care or adopted out. Their Irish mother, who I called 'The Matriarch' but had never met, was severely mentally ill and eventually disappeared back to Ireland to die in a psychiatric home for the elderly.

The life my mother and her sisters had before they were orphaned caused each and every one of them some form of psychological, emotional and physical damage. It was never talked about, but it came up in some way or another when they were older. It seemed that some of their kids had also been affected, including the ones who were put into care when they were babies.

I wanted to know more so called Nat and Marcy again a couple of days later.

It was *so* cool that I could now get to know these two beautiful women again. It was something about the future I had to look forward to. They were the same age as Adult Naomi and didn't smoke weed! I loved that they were related to me and we could be friends. And even if we hadn't been in each other's lives from when we were babies, it was like there was an invisible thread that bonded us to each other that I knew would last a lifetime. Nat and Marcy arrived at just the right time.

Still, talking to them reminded me of the whispered conversations I would overhear between 'The Sisters' when I was little. They kinda had a totally crap time with 'The Matriarch' and I found out that mental illness had coursed through the family tree like an erosive poison. Some of 'The Sisters' had escaped the legacy of mental illness with learning difficulties or addiction issues. Others had suffered the full onslaught, and had ended up institutionalized because of it. Learning this helped me understand a few more things about the bipolar-bear stuff that Adult Naomi had to deal with. It also made me wonder whether this legacy meant we were all, at some point, destined to suffer a mental breakdown, depression, or addiction in our lives. Or was it simply because of what we were told by people around us and the way we were brought up? Either way, it was becoming clearer to me that maybe everything wasn't totally Adult Naomi's fault. Maybe that's why I was here, to figure out how to live a life without it all going mental and feeling like I might wanna kill myself.

But again, why fifteen? I couldn't remember much about being fifteen. One night, when Leo was asleep, I lay on my bed and I tried to remember, but it all felt like a blur. I turned over and saw the red diary lying on the floor. I knew the answer to the question was in that book.

My stomach began to hurt. Those pages gave Adult

Naomi's mind a safe place for all of her innermost thoughts, her secrets. It seemed that the more she wrote year after year, the more she was able to keep those sides of her hidden from view, like a snail crawling into its shell. Adult Naomi didn't want to share, didn't want to be revealed. She was vulnerable, sensitive, and spiritually aware, and her secrets were hidden deep in the pages of her journals.

These new words I had learned – insomnia, depression, mania, listlessness, apathy, detachment – were these the only ways she could survive? And through the diaries I could see that the only people she felt safe to love were Simone and Leo.

It was time. I reached over, picked up the red diary and opened it. I could feel my heart beating. Outside, it began to rain.

Thursday 18 April 1991

This is totally bogus and I am in major shock and I really don't know what the hell to do. I wish I could go back to Liverpool to Dad's and it be Easter all over again cos I sooooo don't wanna be here right now with all this crap going on. I go back to school today to find out that while I was away, ALL – yes, ALL – of my friends have accused the group of boys in our year of sexual assault. What the F**K??? When they told me what happened, I believed them. When you tell a boy to stop, or NO, you don't like where they are putting their hands, then they shouldn't laugh and carry on. But the whole school has turned against my friends and I felt like everyone was watching me to see what I would do, whose side I would choose. We've gone from the most admired to the most

*hated in the space of a week. I was horrified when they
told me, felt like my stomach was eating itself over and
over all day! And now that I'm home, I'm, like, devastated
that this has happened. I am caught in the middle. I tried
to protect my friends from the school, explaining to
everyone their side of the story, but the WHOLE school
thinks they were wrong for telling the teachers. Then I
tried to protect the boys from being expelled and explain
to them where my friends were coming from, that they
went too far and that they should own up to what they
did, but they didn't wanna hear it, saying it was harmless
fun and the girls weren't complaining at the time and
they didn't do anything wrong. I even tried to talk to Mrs
O'Shea but she told me I wasn't there and parents and
THE POLICE were involved and I couldn't do anything
for them! I blame myself, seriously! Why did my dad ask
if we could stay an extra week in Liverpool? Why did
mum say yes? I could have protected the girls. The boys
wouldn't have dared do anything if I was there. Especially
after me kicking Malik's arse in second year when he hit
Simone. The boys know not to mess with me. I feel so bad
for everyone, and kinda angry as well 'cause, like, why the
hell did they go in the classrooms with the boys in the first
place? What were they thinking? If I was there, it wouldn't
have happened. There's nothing I can do, and I feel well
sad about the whole thing. The boys are up in front of the
governors and, like, EVERYONE hates my friends now.
It's all gone really wrong, and I don't know what to do.
Everything's changed and I can't make it right again.
There's no one that can help me make it right again.*

I didn't remember any of this as I was reading it. The page that followed was blank and the next entry was written four days later.

Monday 22 April 1991

We are in hiding. No seriously, we are in hiding. I'm sat on Reece's and Niamh's bunk bed drinking a Cherry B. I'm still in my uniform. Louise has just given me the drink after I asked if my mum was gonna die. Know what she said? 'I really don't know, Nay.' I mean, what the SMEG!!?! I mean, what if she does, like, die? What will we do then? I don't wanna live with my dad. I love him and Marlene but I so don't wanna leave school and my friends. And totally smeggin' wack if they kill my mum. I mean, she didn't do anything wrong.

We have to stay here at Lou's house until it's safe to go home. I mean, it might not be ever. We might have to do another midnight flip and get out of here, if they aren't convinced that my mum didn't steal their drugs. I mean, of course she didn't take their stupid cocaine. My mum is a ganja baby and she likes a drink, everyone knows that, but these horrible men are saying that she and her friend took it and now they want to kidnap her and torture her until she gives it back to them. I mean, like really torture her – we're talking about wires hooked up to car batteries and stuff. God, I mean, she only went to their house for a drink and a spliff and then they came to our house on Friday after school and questioned me, asking me where she was. Bobby B was with them – think he showed them where we lived – and he whispered to me to go inside the

*house and lock the door and not to answer it if the men
came back.*

*Lou said Bobby B told her that they were gonna
kidnap me and keep me until my mum gave them their
drugs back, which she totally has not got, but Bobby B
stopped them.*

*I never listened to him about staying in, though, 'cause
as soon as they left I went to the phone box down the
road and called Mum at work and told her these scary-
looking dudes had come to the house looking for her.
Well, everyone came round to the house. Mum told us to
pack our bags and me and Simone have been here ever
since! I wish Joseph was here; he would know what to do.
But no, he's halfway across the world.*

*I hope my mum doesn't die tonight. She's gone with
Alanson (some big scary-looking gangsta who says he'll
vouch for her) to meet with these drug men to convince
them she didn't take their stupid stuff. I wanna cry but I
can't, but this drink is making me feel a bit better. Please,
please, please, if there is a God up there, please don't let
them kill my mum. I might complain about her all the
time and say I hate her, and she does my head in majorly,
but I do really secretly love her and really don't want
anything bad to happen to her. She's the only mum
I've got!!!*

I felt numb. I could picture my mum's friend Louise's house,
her daughters' bunk bed where I was sitting when I wrote this,
but I had no memory of how scared and desperate I had felt.

I flipped through the pages.

21 November 1991

Just another day at school, although I knew something was different – I woke up feeling weird, you know? Like in a daze. And then when I walked into school Robert Harris turned round to me and wished me Happy Birthday! And then I remembered, shit, I'm sixteen today, and I'd, like, forgotten, but then I realized so had everybody else! Nobody remembered – my dad, my mum, my sister, my friends all forgot. Nobody has celebrated my birth. But you know what? I don't care, I really don't care anymore. It doesn't matter whether I exist or not. I might as well disappear. My friends are totally doing my head in. Joseph has finally left and I don't think he's coming back this time. School is totally wack and I hate devil O'Shea with a passion. My mum is still the Wicked Witch of the West Midlands. Simone is still the·Golden Child! And well, my dad just doesn't seem to care! So why the hell should I?

So I don't feel anything anymore. I just don't care anymore. What's the point?

This was too much for me. I couldn't remember any of it. I closed the diary, shut my eyes and looked deep into my mind, searching for the memory of that entry.

I saw myself still standing outside the house. The door was open and it was time for me to go in, so I pushed it wider and stepped inside. Total darkness. I felt nothing, just the black emptiness of an unoccupied house.

'Hello,' I called out.

I heard nothing, not even an echo of my voice. I knew I had to keep going if I wanted to reach the light. I was afraid, but went in anyway.

As I walked through the large, dark house, I began to see images. Faint images of everything I had seen since I had awoken in the future, images of the small two-bedroom house I shared with Leo and Sophia the cat. Images of my sister and Katie sitting around the table drinking tea. Images of Leo skateboarding and laughing. I felt a mega love for Adult Naomi's family – my family.

I carried on through the darkness, taking deep breaths. I was afraid of what I would find, what I would see, but I couldn't turn back. I needed to find her. I needed to find Adult Naomi. As I walked on, more images played out – of the world and the way it had changed, the way it had seemed to worsen. I saw images of war, melting ice caps, CCTV cameras watching everyone, people protesting, hooded youths rioting, governments ignoring. I didn't like it; the future wasn't meant to turn out like this. I continued on through the darkness, swallowing my fear.

As I passed the rooms of the house I saw the diaries floating around me and an image of me sitting on the floor reading them. Then the image changed to me sitting at the window of a tram, watching the reflection in the window of my school friends and their laughing faces. These faces were replaced by the faces of Adult Naomi's friends. They were smoking and crying. *I don't wanna be stoned anymore. I don't wanna take drugs anymore. There has to be another way*, I thought.

And then the images stopped. I stood still, staring at a large, closed door.

I had known that each step through my mind would lead me to this place. The room contained the answer, the answer to why I had woken up in the future, why I was fifteen years old again. I opened the door.

It was a dark room; the walls were black, almost invisible. I couldn't see the floor, and the ceiling seemed to stretch on forever. The door closed behind me. I stared deeper into the darkness.

'Hello,' I whispered.

I was aware of something flickering. Afraid of what I would see, I turned slowly. A blank screen appeared on the black wall. I heard the familiar whir of a projector and an image appeared. I stopped and watched. It was me, in the bedroom I shared with Simone. I was still in my pyjamas, lying on my Marilyn Monroe duvet, writing an entry in the red diary. I could hear my thoughts echoing around the dark room. I watched and listened.

18 April 1992

Dear diary,

Simone left for Malta yesterday! I hope she has a good time. Wish I was going with them, but my first exam – French – is coming up and I've got to revise for it. I'm crapping myself a bit 'cause I don't think I'm gonna do well in my exams. I thought I would but I've got loads to learn and I haven't even finished my book on Dominique for my Child Development GCSE but Sally says I can spend all day Monday with her so that will be cool. I miss my spars; wonder if they're enjoying their holidays. Even D-Mob's gone caravanning with her dad. Am I, like, the

*only one who never gets to go anywhere? God, the last
holiday we went on was BUTLINS! When I was, like,
nine! My life is so sad! Never been on a plane! I'm the
oldest, I should have gone first, yet Simone (the Golden
Child) gets to go instead! And she's gonna come back all
tanned and gorgeous and I'll still be pale and fat and fed
up! I hate my life, I hate my GCSEs and I hate everything!
I wonder what's on telly tonight . . . So don't know where
Eve is, but I'm gonna see if she can give me some money,
maybe get the new* More *magazine and some chocolate.
I need some new clothes as well. Oh, sack it! I just hate
my life full stop. I wanna be in Malta!*

   *Better get revising, Nay, these smeggin' exams ain't
gonna pass themselves!*

The voice grew quiet, the image disappeared. I stood in
the darkness, in the silence, and then I remembered. It all
came flooding back and I remembered what happened next.
The image appeared again on the other side of me and I saw
it all.

I was lying on my bed writing and then I heard the front
door close and I knew it was my mum. I went downstairs
to say hello but changed my mind because her face was like
thunder. She didn't notice me at first until I asked her about
money and whether I could go out. This seemed to cause some
offence because she freaked out and I just, like, froze on the
spot and watched her face change and twist into a tormented
anger.

She started to shout at me that she had had enough of my
questions, had enough of me.

I exploded. 'What?' I shouted back at her. 'Like, me being here is causing you some form of spaz attack?'

'You have to go,' she shouted and waved her arms at me.

I wanted to storm off upstairs like I normally do but I couldn't move; my legs were stuck and I just stood there and watched her carefully. I was kinda not breathing, hoping she would get lost in her rage and start talking to herself like she sometimes does. Then suddenly something snapped inside me.

'NO! I've had enough of you and I'm sick of hearing about my laziness and bad attitude. I'm frickin' revising for my GCSEs and if you don't like it, well then, that's your problem, 'cause I HAVE TO DO MY EXAMS!!!'

'And then what?' she shouted back.

'What d'ya mean, then what?' I screamed at her.

'What the frig are you going to do after your exams, 'cause you're not staying here anymore?'

Are you kidding me? 'What do you mean? I've got school and my—'

'School's finished! You're not going back to school,' she said.

'But I'm gonna stay on or go to college with my friends.'

'Oh no.' My mum then walked off into the kitchen but I stayed in the living room, totally stunned from what she had just said.

'You're not staying here, fuck that!' she screamed from the kitchen. 'You're not going to college here. You've left school, there's nothing for you here.' She came back to the door, wagging her finger at me.

I sat down on the sofa in shock. I mean, what the smeg? I couldn't stay?

'And what friends? You've got no friends! Where are they? Simone's the one with friends, you haven't friggin' got any!' she shouted.

That was it. I stood up ready for a fight but she bounced through the door back into the kitchen, where she angrily informed the pots and pans that I was a lazy bastard, I had no friends and no life and I wasn't staying in her house any longer.

I was speechless. I mean, totally in shock. I mean, all's I wanted was some pocket money and it ended with the reality that as soon as my exams were over, I totally had to find somewhere else to live because I was no longer wanted in the house. Hell, even in the town.

Holding back the tears, I went back into the kitchen. 'But where am I supposed to go? I've got nowhere to go.'

She turned to me. 'What are you on about? You can go live with your dad. He can have you now.'

'My frickin' dad?' I screamed. 'No way, Jose!' I shook my head, as if that would shake the reality of moving to Liverpool right out of me.

And then she went crazy on me. The shouts and screams got louder; the words were mouthed more slowly. Everything just got more hurtful. It was mental. I didn't understand, and then everything just went blurry and I blanked out the rest of what she was saying.

In the dark room I took a step back from the image.

I remembered. I remembered what it had felt like that day seventeen years ago.

The image played on.

And that's when she dropped the final bomb. 'I mean, what's the fucking point of you?' she screamed.

'What?' I stumbled back through the door. Did she just ask me what was the point of me? Did my mother just question my whole existence?

And that's when I realized she already knew I was going to live with Art, that she had decided that before she had even started. *What's the point of me? Like, why the hell am I here? I* thought. *What's my purpose?*

I opened my mouth to answer her, but I think the look on my face must have jolted her out of her angry place and told her she had gone too far, as she always did. Her face seemed to morph into a strange mix of righteous indignation, scornful sorrow and regret. I was seriously trying to fight back the tears. I was *majorly* angry, though. I mean, how could she say such bogus things? I stood there trying to figure out what had I done to deserve this? She'd sent my sister on a fabulous beach holiday and then, like, gone and attacked my very existence the next day.

'I HATE YOU SO MUCH!' I screamed at her and ran upstairs to my bedroom. I slammed the door as hard as I could, threw myself on my bed and burst into tears.

All I could think of was *that* question: *What's the point of you?*

After a while, the tears stopped and I figured it out. *I don't know why I am here, so I've got no point, right?* I asked myself. *And if there is no point to me, I might as well not exist, right? I'm gonna fail my exams, I'm gonna fail at life. I am a failure.*

After a while I heard the front door slam shut. Eve had left.

I felt so alone but could see it all clearly. There was no point to me. I totally didn't matter and maybe I shouldn't have even been born.

I knew that there was only one answer to my problem.

I got off my bed, went into my mum's room and found a small brown bottle of white pills in the top cupboard of her wardrobe and threw as many as I could down my throat while drinking the tap water from the bathroom sink. I just wanted it over as quickly as possible. I didn't care about anybody or anything else. I didn't think about a note, or who would find me, or even why I was doing it. I just wanted it ALL over. I wanted to stop that voice in my head from taunting me, teasing me about my bogus life. I was fat and ugly and nobody was bothered whether I lived or died. I wanted the pain to stop.

If my family don't even remember my birthday, or drug dealers wanna kidnap me, or boys wanna sexually assault my friends and I can't protect them, then I don't matter, how I feel doesn't matter, so then they won't miss me when I'm dead, I thought as I drank the water.

I burst into tears again. I had no control over anything but I knew I had control over the amount of drugs I could get in me before the pain became too much. So I swallowed as many as I could and lay on my mum's bed. It stopped the tears and all of those crap questions eventually faded into the background. It was like I was surrounded by a fog of peace, and my breathing slowed and I felt calm. It felt right. I closed my eyes. I really thought it was time for me to go.

I took a step back from the image and took a deep breath; it was all too much. It was as if the house in my mind knew how I felt because, like with the image that had played before, I heard a voice again. My voice, echoing in the darkness, telling me what had happened the day I had tried to kill myself. I turned and saw myself lying still on the bed. I was sleeping. I looked peaceful.

BAM!

The front door slammed shut and I jumped up out of this semi-conscious state. It was dark outside so I must have fallen asleep. I knew my mum was back and I had to get out of her room, but when I jumped up off her bed my legs went all spazmode on me and I fell to the floor and whacked my head on the door frame. It mashed me up; my head felt strange, I couldn't get my brain to tell my legs to walk and I knew if she caught me, she would kill me.

'What are you doing?' she shouted up at me from the bottom of the stairs.

'Nothing.' I tried to give her serious attitude but I sounded kinda drunk.

I used the door frame to pull myself up from the floor and then I felt majorly scared. She had come back too early. I was supposed to be dead. And then something weird happened. I got to the bathroom and stood there just staring at my reflection in the mirror, and I looked like a stranger. It was me, but the older version of me; I didn't recognize myself. My head was hurting and my heart was beating really fast.

And then it was like a switch flipped in my brain and I just knew. In that second, in the bathroom, on my own staring at this face in the mirror, I couldn't do it. I knew I had a place, somewhere. I just had to find it. I didn't want to die. I just needed some time to find where I belonged. To find a point. I just needed help.

So I splashed my face with cold water a few times and stuck my fingers down my throat. It tasted rank but I kept saying, 'Get a grip, Nay, you smeg,' until it became my motto for staying alive and I couldn't throw up anymore. I knew then that I had to tell Eve, there was no choice. I didn't know what I had taken and could have needed the hospital. I thought after what had happened that morning that she would be feeling mega amounts of guiltiness and would understand why I had reacted the way I did and get me to A&E post haste. I would throw up properly; she would apologise, realize she had made a mistake and allow me to continue on with my plans to stay home. *So* wrong!

I slowly walked downstairs and into the living room, where she was stood by the coffee table staring out through the window. I looked but couldn't see what she was looking at.

'Mum, I've just taken some tablets but threw up.'

'What?' She spun around and the look of horror on her face as the colour slowly drained from her skin made me feel well bad for what I had done.

'Where from?' she shouted angrily.

'From the top of your wardrobe,' I told her, and then she grabbed me by my hair. I tried to pull her hands away but the more I tried, the tighter she held on. She then proceeded to swing my frickin' skull back and forth with one hand while slapping me upside the head with the other, all the while screaming unintelligible words at me.

The rest was a blur. My hair still in her hands, she pulled me out of the house, shouting at me all the way to the corner shop.

When we got to the shop, Happy Shopper Harry was stood behind the counter concentrating on something. He was kinda like a pretend uncle – well, he used to let my mum get cigs and milk from his back door when the shop was closed on a Sunday and we played with his daughter until she grew up and went to Camp America, and he would always listen to you, no matter what was wrong or what you had done. Happy Shopper Harry's shop was the only one we never nicked from when we were kids; he was top bananas. Mum told him what I had done.

'Oh, Naomi.' He looked at me over his glasses, a look of pity on his face, and shook his head. 'Why?'

My mum was on the verge of tears. 'Because she's bloody stupid, that's why.'

I was mortified and just hung my head down in embarrass-mental shame while Harry served my mum with two cans of her lager and some cigarettes.

'Bloody suicide! Her dad would kill me if she bloody kills herself,' Mum said, looking for some money in her purse.

I wanted to cry, like, right there and then. I still couldn't believe it!

'Do you want a lift to the hospital, Eve?' he asked my mum. 'I can get Betty to take over.'

Please, no, I thought. I shook my head at him. The thought of anyone else knowing made me wish I had really died.

'No, it's okay, she'll be fine,' my mum said as she left the shop. I followed behind her. She was still screaming stuff at me until we got to our neighbour Thelma's house. I had to sit there in Thelma's living room while Thelma, Joanne and Carol just frickin' sat there staring at me, biting their lips nervously as Eve told them what I had just done. Again, the looks of horror and pity mirrored Harry's and I hung my head down.

'Don't you think she should go to the hospital, Eve?' Thelma asked, most probably not wanting her neighbour's daughter dropping dead in her living room or herself becoming an accessory to murder.

'No, she can sit there and suffer; she won't die.' My mum pulled the ring off the can of lager and gulped it down. The drunken feeling I'd had was gone; I was shaking and sobbing and felt so full of this, like, major frickin' soul-crushing shame that I just couldn't look at anyone.

18 April 1992 (same night)

I've got to keep writing. If I keep writing, then I'll stay awake and maybe I won't die. I can't believe what I've done. I didn't mean to, it just happened. I didn't mean for it to go so far, but I didn't know what else to do and as soon as I did it I told Eve, but she went ballistic – I mean, all-out warfare, man – and I don't know what to do, 'cause she's still in Thelma's drinking and what if I die?

I mean, Thelma helped me; well, she went into her kitchen and poured me a glass of water and made me a slice of toast. By this time I was just drained and exhausted and I couldn't keep my eyes open, I just wanted to sleep, but I couldn't tell if it was the tablets or everything that had happened so I ate the toast. It tasted like cardboard and I drank the water and did my best to hide my surprise when I tasted salt in it. I looked at Thelma and she gave me a wink. Eve was deep in conversation so I asked if I could use the toilet and went into the bathroom at the back of the house. I stood over the toilet and gulped the salt water down in one and stuck my fingers down my throat again and threw up the toast and this white acidy stuff.

I just wanted to leave after that. I wanted to come home. My stomach must be empty of the tablets so I'm sure I won't die. Eve said I could come home.

You know what? I felt so free when I left that house, like a caged bird that had been let out and had found a crack open in a forgotten window and escaped. I found my way straight here to my bed and I'm curled up under my duvet, with my feet wrapped in it at the bottom 'cause I'm cold and I feel sick. I genuinely thought Eve was waiting to see if I passed out first, then she would have taken me to hospital. Why didn't she take me to the hospital? Didn't she believe me? Did she think I was lying? Maybe it wasn't serious enough, or maybe she just doesn't care. I hate her so much.

Still, I'm lying here writing this, crying and praying. Please, if there is anyone out there listening, I don't want to die, and if you could at all help it, can you make sure I don't die? Because I think I know the answer to my problem. I won't know the point of me, I won't know why I am here until I get as far away as possible from Eve! Far away from here.

Just please don't let me die and I'll never take another drug again, not even a painkiller.

And then maybe one day, everything will be okay.
Maybe.

Naomi x

I closed my eyes and the images, the memories playing out in the house in my mind stopped. It had all now become clear and for the first time I actually had some flashes of memory from my near future. That night had been the start of my drug-taking journey. It was me; I didn't matter, so my life didn't matter and I had allowed it to spiral out of control from then on. I remembered I started to smoke weed, I failed my exams, I even went into an exam stoned one day, and then I started to take harder drugs.

I did exactly what Adult Naomi had done. *I* got stuck and split, left the building, possibly the house of *my* mind.

When I was fifteen, *I* split. Just like when Little Naomi was six and was raped and when Adult Naomi was twenty-nine and fell down the stairs. It happened to me too when I was fifteen and couldn't cope with school and the possibility of my mum dying and then I did it again when I was sixteen when I tried to kill myself. *I* split.

But I think I got stuck at fifteen; my mind stayed fifteen because of that time with my dad during the Easter holidays, when he bought us loads of chocolate eggs and took us for meals in nice restaurants. He took us on shopping sprees; bought us loads and told us over and over how much he loved us. That was the last time I felt like a child, the last time I felt safe, protected.

And then everything went terribly, horribly wrong.

And I split.

I then remembered I had a fight with my school friend Katie, a physical fist fight. I attacked her because people had been telling me she had been talking about me. She hit me back and I bit her head with my braces on. She was devastated. I was numb. I am remembering it.

And I split.

I tried to cope with everything and started to somehow separate from my reality. I wanted so much to feel like a child again, feel protected. Except that ended the day I was told I had to leave. I had to face being sixteen and the fact that I was truly on my own; to fend for myself in a world I had no clue about. I couldn't cope so I tried to kill myself. That didn't work, so I turned to drugs.

And I split.

The threats from the cocaine men to kill my mum; my friends and the sexual assault and not being able to protect them; failing my exams; not wanting to leave school, but hating it at the same time. In the space of a year, everything fell apart. Joseph and my mum were splitting up and I remembered that – as great as our Easter visit in Liverpool was – I would wake up in the middle of the night to hear my dad and Marlene arguing. Simone seemed to be protected from it all, and I, like a sponge, absorbed it all and eventually my mind split.

It went wrong and I wanted to stay, no, needed to be somewhere where it felt safe. I needed the pain to stop. I couldn't find anywhere.

Eventually, death was my only answer; if not death, then drugs.

And my mind split.

I turned from the images in the darkness and saw a small orange light floating in front of me. I reached my hand out and grabbed hold of it, carrying it through the house until I reached the very window I had spent almost six weeks staring into, locked outside. This time, I was staring out of it, from the inside.

The street was still dark. I placed the light on the window-sill and caught my reflection in the glass.

I knew then why I had woken up in the future: it was me. It had all started with me. I had got stuck, stuck in a time when I had given up on myself. When I felt that I really didn't matter. And the small part of me that still believed I did, I cut out of my mind and buried with drugs. No wonder my life had turned out the way it had. The amount of bad stuff I had gone through before I was sixteen . . . no wonder I didn't wanna grow up. The only way my mind could cope was to break itself into pieces and hide those pieces away in the pages of my diaries and deep in the darkness of my mind, in the darkness of a house.

Everything that had happened to me, up until that age, had proved to me that there was no hope, no hope for a better future, no hope for me. In the end, when things got really bad, that's where my mind would go, to the safety and the security that thoughts of my death would bring. It would mean peace instead of pain.

I looked at my reflection in the window. My face changed into hers, into Adult Naomi's. 'I am so sorry,' I sobbed to her.

The pain pulled my mind out of the dark house.

I opened my eyes, got off the bed, and looked out of the window into the night sky. Rain was falling and I stared hard through the wavy patterns it created under the street light. The salt from my tears stung my face. I took a deep breath, my heart shrank in my chest, and I cried.

Remembering had eventually led me to this point; it was a wound so heavy with pain that it forced its way through me and pulled me into a cold darkness. I choked through the tears. I felt weak and my lungs ached.

Neither the world nor my life had turned out the way they were supposed to and after spending several weeks reading my diaries, I had realized why.

I could see clearly now, the constant running away and drifting from place to place, smoking weed and taking drugs. Over the weeks, I had read in the diaries that Adult Naomi had dealt with a drug-addicted boyfriend, emotionally abusive relationships, being a single mother, running her own businesses, teaching others how to heal while trying to heal herself, a cocaine habit, a drug-induced breakdown . . . She had been declared bankrupt, lost all of her possessions, been homeless, and in effect had to start again . . .

And then I woke up.

Because it all began with me, Teen Nay, and ended with Adult Naomi's future. I sobbed as I thought about everything I had read from start to finish, the last seventeen years of Adult Naomi's life – no, *my life* – in a nutshell. All of it led to this future, the council house, the cat and the car and the son who looked like her. A future where Adult Naomi tried to find some stability, some safety and security, but always felt like she failed.

And all because I had buried me, hiding behind a facade of smiles. A mask, like the one Leo had made me. That told the outside world that everything was okay, that everything was all glittery and gold, when really inside I was breaking. Constantly breaking down.

I turned my head into the pillow and screamed. I screamed so terrifyingly loud that I was surprised Leo didn't wake up. The released emotion welled up like a giant wave crashing against me with such a force, my body repelled it in droves. I threw up in the bin and screamed with rage, with anger at Eve, at Art, at the cocaine men, at the men who abused me, at the women in Thelma's house. I screamed at the world for letting me down, at myself for allowing this to happen. For playing a part in the death of me. My head wanted to explode, but I couldn't cry quickly enough. I curled my body into the foetal position and lay there on my bed for what felt like an eternity, and I cried out every pain, every heartbreak, everything I had ever done to myself.

The room grew dark. I felt empty, numb; my head pounded into my swollen face. I didn't want to move; I had given up and nothing was going to pull me out. I had started the destruction of my life and no matter how hard she had tried, Adult Naomi just couldn't put it back together.

Somewhere in the darkness of my mind, I heard a faint whisper, a gentle voice telling me to breathe. I took a deep breath and eventually the tears stopped. The pain subsided. I had cried myself into exhaustion. I closed my eyes and stared into the darkness that had once housed all of those memories. I saw nothing. 'I'm scared,' I whimpered to the empty bedroom. I searched for some hope – that same small hope I'd had lying in my bed thinking I was dying seventeen years ago. I looked into the darkness and saw me lying in the bed again, under the Marilyn Monroe duvet cover, crying, praying I wouldn't die. I had heard the gentle whisper of a voice, telling me to breathe. Now, lying in Adult Naomi's bed seventeen years later, I heard that same voice again.

'Breathe, Naomi, breathe,' it said.

As I drifted off and fell into a deep sleep, it gently whispered again. A song, like a lullaby, singing the words, 'Sleep. You know who you are, everything is well within. We love you, you are protected. Sleep.'

Protected?

10

The Scorpion Queen

The more and more each is impelled by that which is intuitive,
or the relying upon the soul force within,
the greater, the farther,
the deeper, the broader,
the more constructive may be the result.

EDGAR CAYCE

Something has changed, I thought, as I opened my eyes the next morning.

I climbed off the bed and opened the curtains. The sun was shining and the sky was a beautiful cornflower blue peppered with dashes of white cloud. Everything looked different. I opened the window, breathed in the city air – a faint mix of car fumes and freshly cut grass from the park – and listened to the birds singing the new day in. The tall evergreens stood opposite, proud and protective like giant guards watching over me. I could sense this universal agreement that I was okay and that all would be well in my world.

Yes, something had changed. I was still a teenager and I

was still in the future. But somewhere inside of me, I knew I had the power to handle it. I knew that I was going to make things different, that I was going to change things and that this life was going to get much, much better.

'I have to go away!' I shouted to the awakening street.

I turned around to the messy, undecorated room. 'But before I go, I'm so going to decorate you. In fact, I'm going to do the whole house and get rid of that puke salmon colour downstairs.'

In the mirror, I looked at my puffy face. My eyes were still swollen but I stared at my body, my skin, my hair and opened my mouth to flash my teeth. They were stained by years of coffee and smoking. 'And I am going to get you all sorted,' I said to the reflection, whilst doing a three-hundred-and-sixty-degree turn. 'This body, my body. All of you.'

I ran a bath and, whilst the tub filled, I tidied the bedroom, removing every diary from the floor. The red diary had served its purpose and I knew it was time to put it away for good. Leaving out the 2008 diary, I packed the rest into a box and sealed it with Sellotape, promising myself I would never open it again. I didn't have to; the diaries had given me what I'd needed – a past I had to know but was now ready to forget. Even though I understood Adult Naomi more and could see that it was me who had started her on this path, all that mattered to me was the present and the decisions I could make in that moment to turn her future – no, *my* future – into the one I deserved. In spite of everything, I reckoned that holiday I never got didn't matter anymore, because I was going to take myself on one.

'Egypt!' I exclaimed to my sister later that day.

'Wow, really? Egypt? Are you sure?' she questioned.

'Absolutely.' I knew she would be concerned and I knew I would have to convince her I would be okay to go on my own. From conversations with Katie and Simone, I had learned that Adult Naomi *had* in fact visited all of the places on the postcards on the kitchen wall. She and Leo had taken a few holidays. He had even gone to Canada with his father, which I was surprised by. I still didn't want to meet him, though. Adult Naomi had felt betrayed by him too many times and I felt I needed to protect her from his lack of respect and loyalty.

But in one diary, she had spoken a lot about Ancient Egypt, Kemetic wisdom, and something called Hermetic philosophy. They sounded like they belonged on *The Muppet Show* but hey, I believed I owed it to her to get there.

Once I explained this to my sister, googled where I'd be staying so I could show her and convinced her how safe I would be, she agreed that it was maybe what I needed and said she would take care of Leo while I was gone. It turned out Adult Naomi had saved quite a bit of money, so I could afford to go. My passport said I was thirty-two, so no one would know I was fifteen, and being the sensible teenager I was, I reassured her that there was no chance of me wandering off with strangers (ahem). I trusted myself and so did Simone and that's all that was needed for me to find a suitcase and book the holiday.

And then in a totally weird way, I began to remember. It was almost like the belief that I could make things better had allowed my mind to relax more. The more it relaxed, the more memories started to drip-feed into my mind, like a leaky tap slowly filling a plugged sink. With the help of Simone and Adult Naomi's friends I began to remember. And what was majorly wigged was that I was the one in control of it all.

The more I remembered, the closer I felt to Adult Naomi and the more protective I became of her. She still hadn't returned and that was okay too. She had been through some mega hard times. We both had, but she had relied on smeg-head people, been betrayed by Jekyll friends, been attacked and lied to by those she trusted, and yet she still believed in love and had a compassion for people that I totally didn't get, but kind of respected at the same time.

Dean reminded me of the time he and Adult Naomi had gone to a small festival together and the organizers were so off their faces, she had taken over the barn where they were making breakfasts and cooked for almost everyone there. As he told me this, I had a kinda flashback/flashforward to jumping up and down on a trampoline whilst on magic mushrooms, giggling uncontrollably. Weird!

Katie reminded me of the times Adult Naomi had sat with her sons and helped them with their homework and supported them through their exams. I had another kind of flashback/flashforward of trying to figure out algebra with her eldest.

An Alanis Morissette song brought back images of me pushing a 9lb 9 baby out of my . . . well, I won't go there, but it was in a birthing pool while Simone, Simone's best friend Lynette and Leo's father held my hands and told me to push.

I also remembered early bits about Leo's dad. Yeah, kinda

intense and a bit rank, actually. He had kids from other relationships and was seriously commitment shy. Trying to relate to him while she was pregnant was STRESSFUL!

And then I remembered having sex! Which was totally mentally bizarro since I was still a virgin. During a TV episode of *Angel*, I flashbacked/flashforwarded to an ex-boyfriend dressed in a long black leather coat, who was tall with dark, brooding good looks and who Adult Naomi really liked and had a lot of fun with.

Some memories weren't so pleasant – people getting shot, friends being raped, heated arguments and fights in clubs – but I somehow managed to steer them away, like a politician avoiding embarrassing questions.

I also started to get the whole pet thing and one day decided to stroke Sophia and explain to her what was going on. I didn't sneeze and she didn't seem to care that I wasn't Adult Naomi; she just seemed to want to be around me anyway. Which I kinda liked.

And so that's how it was: music, food, images, clothes, smells, words, all sparked memories of a rich past, of experiences that played out like a film on the projector of my mind. But as it was Adult Naomi's past and my future, the emotions attached to those images were not mine, so I wasn't attached to them. I felt them, I acknowledged what or who they were about, and I just moved on to the next image with, like, this aloof curiosity.

As I began to remember, I wrote more stuff in Adult Naomi's diary.

27 June 2008

Dear Adult Naomi,

I wanted to let you know that while I am here, I am only going to speak to the people I want to and will happily avoid the calls of those I don't. I just don't get your friends, sorry. I mean, Dean is way cool and Katie is top bananas, but the rest of them? And anyway, I'm still well impressed with the call-screening thingy on a mobile phone, so I pretend I haven't received text messages and then switch my phone off until I want to speak to someone and then I switch it back on. I'm telling you this because I think it's important you know that those someones are mainly family, including our cousins Nat and Marcy, who are, like, really safe and our age and so should be our friends!

Got in touch with Dad this week. Even though he's used to you going incommunicado for months on end, he was happy to hear from me. I told him what had happened; he went very quiet and then asked me did I wanna go the hospital, but I told him no frickin' way! The last thing you need is ignoramus psycho doctors like that Dr (dick) Davies that can't help you. I told him this and then he said as long as I was okay and that he would come and stay and help me decorate the bedroom. Do you like it? The paint is called Hollywood, and wow, IKEA is, like, wicked!!!

He came to stay at the weekend and helped me decorate. I cried when I saw him, not because he had aged – in fact, he hardly looks any different. He has a

*little pot belly and a couple of grey hairs in his stubble
but he is still my dad. I had missed him. And I kind of get
it. I found out Eve told Simone to leave home a year after
me and go and live with Art as well. Maybe her forcing
us to go and live with him wasn't a bad thing in the end.
I wouldn't have ended up in Manchester, and I wouldn't
have had Leo. And Art has been a great dad to Leo as
well. So, bonus! But he likes to talk to me a lot about
politics and stuff, which is totally weird 'cause he's treating
me like an adult!*

*Oh. My. Dayz. JJ!!! I screamed, cried, and laughed
all at once when I saw him for the first time ever. No way
have we got a brother! He's like this really tall, lighter-
skinned genetic hybrid of me, Simone, Leo and Art; he
has the dimples, the cheekbones, the almond-shaped
brown eyes that disappear when he smiles. Sooooo
freaky! The only difference is he's skinny (didn't get the fat
gene then) and he's got a mop of golden brown curls. I
know you know this but writing it down is kind of helping
me remember stuff. He speaks really posh (Sim says his
mum is posh) and he knows A LOT for his age. In fact, I
suspect he is somewhat of a prodigy ('Everybody is in tha
place' . . . remember that tune?) Anyway, I was a little
wary at first; he and Simone seemed to get on so well
and I wasn't sure of your relationship with him, until he
mentioned films and sci-fi in the same sentence. That
was it, we spent the whole weekend watching your sci-fi
collection and I introduced him to the 'greats': Blade
Runner, Logan's Run and the first three Star Wars*

episodes (which are the last three). He showed me The
Matrix *(wow!), the* Terminator *films and the last three
episodes of* Star Wars *(which are the first three)! I showed
him* Red Dwarf *as well. So me and JJ have bonded over a
love of film and I am glad Art let go of his hatred of 'Tory
toffs and all of their offspring' long enough to procreate
once more and produce our gorgeous, talented and
extremely smart brother.*

*I think it's time to contact Joseph's brood! I miss my
stepbrothers and sisters!*

I hope you're okay, wherever you are.

    Love,

      Teen Nay x

And I did. I spoke to all seven of them. I saved the best till
last.

Maxine was four years younger than me and we were very
close as children. We shared a birthday and out of all my stepbrothers and sisters, she was the one I got on with the most
and seemed to have remained close to in adult life. In my
mind, the last time we had spoken, she was eleven years of
age. I couldn't believe she was twenty-eight now.

'MAXI–PAD!' I screamed down the phone – my loving
nickname for her. Yeah, a sanitary towel, but hey, she still
loved me!

'Oh my God, no one has called me that for years!' she
laughed.

'Oh my dayz, you sound OLD!' I said, startled by her voice.
'Has Sim told you what's happened to me then?'

She hadn't, so Maxine listened in stunned silence as I told

her of everything that had happened over the past couple of months.

'Bloody 'ell, Nay. What ya gonna do now?' she asked me.

'Chipping to Egypt.'

'Wow, seriously?'

'Yeah, it's been mental, I *sooooo* need a holiday.'

'Are you sure you'll be all right going on your own?' It was weird, my eleven-year-old sister worrying about me.

'I will be safe, sorted, don't worry, sis; everything is under control,' I said confidently.

'Well, call me when you land. Let me know you get there okay.'

'I will.'

'Promise?'

'I smeg you not, I will call.'

She started to laugh again. 'Smeg,' she sniggered. 'What's a fridge got to do with it?'

'A what?' I had no clue what she was talking about until Maxine gave me the Smeg-is-now-the-name-of-a-fridge-maker's-and-not-a-cool-swear-word explanation and also told me *again* how my beloved Lister had ended up in *Coronation Street*. The first time around I hadn't really taken it in, but now I couldn't hide the disappointment I felt in my hero and vowed to never use the word 'smeg' again. Maxine found this hilarious. I did not; I was still getting over the death of Kurt Cobain.

So after spending time with those I loved and reconnecting with the friends I liked, a sense of balance came to everything that had been messed up. I was as happy and as settled as I could be and the connection I felt with those around me brought me closer to Adult Naomi. I kinda stopped wanting to go back to 1992 and instead decided to fill the future with experiences that were mine.

I never wanted to smoke again. So I exercised by walking and doing a bit of jogging around the local park. This kept the desire to get stoned at bay so I got Adult Naomi's sachet of weed from the bedside drawer and threw it away.

As my brain began to change, so did my taste buds. I found that my digestive system just couldn't handle dairy products and eventually I gave up the cottage cheese. And one morning, after a late night with Dean and some pear cider, I found myself craving a cup of hot black coffee.

Several days later, I packed a large suitcase and charged up the iPod, which still blew my frickin' mind. (When Simone showed me a camera that took pictures you could actually see on a screen and were saved on a chip – no fish in sight – I almost hit the deck in complete major shock!) Everyone was so supportive of me having a holiday. So on the day I left, I gave Simone and Leo a mega hug and while heading to the airport thought for the first time, *I'm starting to like the future.*

As my plane passed over the deserts of North Africa, I felt a subtle interior shift. The warmth of the sun shone through the small window and the curves and dips of the sand beneath me seemed to move like gentle waves on a golden sea. It took my breath away and I instantly felt connected to the earth below. I felt like a travelling child, who had left home years ago, but now, older and wiser, was coming back. This country had been waiting patiently for me with open arms, welcoming me back. I couldn't shake the feeling that I had been here before and that I belonged.

Major déjà vu!

The plane landed at Marsa Alam in the early evening. As soon as I stepped onto the tarmac the waning sun shone down, warming up every cell in my body. I knew at once that I'd made the right decision in coming here.

Marsa Alam, an isolated fishing village, was situated on the south-western coast of the Red Sea. The few resorts built along the rich blue coastline were small and the nearest city was four hours away. As our coach turned the corner into the hotel car park, I noticed a man sitting outside one of the hotel shops on a small stool, smoking a cigarette. He watched the coach pull up through squinted eyes, which seemed to, like, give him a permanent smile on his old face. I smiled at him. He laughed and nodded his head. I had no clue what he found so funny, but I laughed with him anyway.

Once in the hotel, our holiday rep, Mark – a very friendly and very camp guy – welcomed our group, which was full of couples, a few foges and this young couple from Leeds, who I chatted to on the coach and who seemed nice when I asked them to take a picture of me when we arrived. It was kind of a quiet group, which suited me fine. I missed the start of Mark's speech, as I was too busy staring at his hair, which had been Brylcreemed to within an inch of its life. It sat on top of his head like a shiny black wave captured in mid-air. Mark was to be our 'go-to guy' if we needed anything or had any problems with the hotel. I was counting on having a very problem-free, STRESS-FREE stay, so reckoned on not seeing Mark at all.

I felt so relaxed that even when he informed us our rooms weren't ready, I was happy to wait.

The setting sun was disappearing behind the hotel rooms into a distant royal-blue sea but it still shone, reddish and orange, over everything in the opulent lobby. In the centre, there was a raised circular marble platform, flagged by four pillars; golden rails fenced in a square around it, leaving a gap for access. I decided it was a good place to sit, so I walked up the two marble steps and sat on one of the half-moon-shaped blue sofas. Though it was situated in the centre of the hotel lobby, sitting there seemed to separate me from everyone else. My gaze eventually landed on this humongous russet bronze bird. I hadn't noticed it before because it was placed at the highest point of the room on the wall above the reception desk.

It was a phoenix and seeing it made me suddenly remember something.

I pulled out Adult Naomi's diary and started to write.

Dear Adult Naomi,

I just quickly wanted to write to you while I am waiting for my hotel room key. We are so meant to be here! There's a huge phoenix on the wall and it's carrying a massive golden orb in its claws, and its feathers are trailing all curly behind it. It's beautiful, magnificent, like a god watching over its children playing; it feels like it's watching over the room protectively. It just made me remember. Remember when mum let me have that Christmas party? I think she felt mega guilty 'cause she

*had forgotten my sixteenth birthday! Remember Robert
Harris got drunk and threw up over the front garden
wall and my girl Foxy and her mad boyfriend Billy
were kissing on my top bunk bed and everyone went
on for weeks about how it was a wicked party? I kinda
remember how great I felt – even though I had to leave
Wolverhampton, I went out in style; I felt good about
myself for a while. Remember? And remember how much
we were into star signs and astrology? We used to sell
horoscopes to the kids in school. I totally loved being a
Scorpio, remember? Mysterious, secretive, but sexy and
smart, that was stuff I thought about myself – no, think
about myself – and made me look forward to being a
woman, throwing great parties, people liking being
around me and stuff, but you don't feel like that anymore,
which has made me well sad. But the Phoenix bird, I
remember now, it's like, the original symbol for the
scorpion. I am taking it as a reminder or a sign from the
universe (as you put it) that I have chosen the right place.
We are so meant to be here!*

    Love,

        Teen 'too sexy for your car' Nay x

Humming the Right Said Fred song that my friends and
I used to dance around to provocatively, I took in the rest of
the decor. My jaw almost hit the floor when I saw what was
above me. Sat atop of the four pillars was a dome, the inside of
which was painted white with seven golden stars. Underneath
the stars was a ring of symbols, which on closer inspection, I
realized were the twelve signs of the zodiac, and I was sitting

directly underneath the scorpion sign. I sat and stared in disbelief – had I been *expected*?

As I stared at the zodiac signs from Aquarius through to Capricorn, I got the sudden feeling I was being watched, like someone's eyes were piercing right through me. I was right. The same man who'd been sitting outside the shop earlier was standing in the shadow of the entrance, watching me as a young bellboy chatted to him animatedly. It took a while for it to register, but once I figured I must have looked a bit tapped sitting there, mouth wide open as I stared up at the ceiling, I looked away. When I looked up again the man had gone.

Moments later, we were handed keys and Mark led us to the rooms, which were dotted around the complex in separate two-up, two-down apartments. The outside walls were a red colour, others terracotta, and they looked as if someone had taken a chisel from the gods and carved them out of the rock face. I felt like I was in a North African version of Bedrock and expected a Bedouin Fred Flintstone to walk past, waving and shouting, 'Yabba dabba doooooo! Have a great time!'

Mark led me up a set of stone steps to the top floor, where he showed me into my room. It smelled of warm jasmine flowers.

'Right, darrrrrling.' He swung an arm around dramatically. 'This is yours; it has a separate bathroom, a double bedroom and a separate dressing room.' He handed me a file. 'Here's your welcome pack. My number is in there; call me day or night if you need anything, sweetie.' He almost skipped to the door, then swivelled on his feet. 'Someone will bring your suitcase up soon,' he said happily. And then he was gone.

I explored properly. My bathroom was white marble tiled

and spacious. Next to this was a separate dressing room. Built from a green malachite stone, with black and ochre marble walls, it had a walk-in wardrobe, a dressing table with mirror and a small wicker sofa with green cushions. A small window with spotlights looked into the double bedroom; it was like a cross between Egyptian art deco and a scene from a 1930s Hollywood movie and I loved every single part of it.

My large double room consisted of a queen-sized bed flanked either side by small wooden cabinets and large black lamps. A sofa sat in the far corner, which looked out through the patio doors, and opposite it sat a black wooden cabinet desk with TV, phone and lamp. This was going to be my home for the next nine days. It felt like a sanctuary already and was just enough for me.

I opened the doors onto the balcony and the sight and smell of the lush green lawns and the pink and orange flowers totally took my breath away. The hotel's gardeners were watering the plants. Some of them looked up and smiled at me. I smiled back. Beyond the garden was a beautiful secluded golden sandy beach on which tall palm trees stood, shading sun loungers and wooden umbrellas. It was paradise. I watched as the African sun dipped into the sea, bidding farewell to the day and making way for the stars. One by one, they appeared in the sky as if someone had flicked a switch on, ready for the darkness.

A knock on the door jolted me from my trance. A man dressed in the cream hotel uniform stood holding my suitcase. As I opened the door wider he gave me the most gorgeous smile. He was major fitness! He had soft, smooth skin, high cheekbones, a chiselled jaw and those Colgate advert white teeth. His eyes sparkled mischievously and his straight jet-black hair curled at the edges. He looked as if he belonged on the cover of Arabic *Vogue* or something, not in a hotel at the end of the Red Sea. I stood staring at him for a second too long, then felt like a total spaz and giggled instead. He laughed at me.

I fumbled in my purse and gave him ten Egyptian dollars.

'My name is Ahmed.' His voice was deep. 'If you need anything from me, you call housekeeping and I will be here straight away.'

My skin burned red. 'Th . . . th . . . thanks,' I stuttered. My mouth was dry.

He gave me another gorgeous sexy smile, and before my knees totally went and I wrapped up on the floor, he left.

I went back out to the balcony for some air and to stop my embarrassmental shame and, in that moment, I knew without a doubt that Egypt was going to be just what I needed to get over waking up in the future. It had been a long day, though, so to the soundtrack of the waves gently lapping against the beach, I came back in to settle myself into my room. I unpacked, had a shower and got in my PJs. I was in bed moments later and picking up the 2008 diary. I flipped open the first entry Adult Naomi had written earlier in the year. It was all about the circle of life – or hakuna matata as Leo would say – and energy.

13 January 2008

This came to me when I meditated tonight.
The energy we possess flows from the divine soul.
The divine soul is all that has been, is, and ever will be.

*Energy moves through our souls to the physical body
and back out to the universe as a vibration, eventually
returning to the divine soul. This continuous figure
of eight rhythm mirrors the law of contraction and
expansion which governs the cosmos. When this takes
shape and form in our lives and we see it, we know it is
the divine consciousness manifesting and is in everything,
no matter what it is. It is ALL that exists, manifesting
through different vibrations into this world and those
vibrations are given names. Like a flower: it's born in
spring, it blossoms in summer, it decays in autumn and
after winter it is destined to return to the earth. We are
that flower. We come from pure divine spirit into a
physical body and then leave our physical state to return
to pure spirit. This is the journey of creation, the cosmic
journey of the soul. This constant creation of ourselves
through the experience of energy is so that we know the
true essence of who we are. The true you within. Then
and only then will we know our true vibration. Our
true name.*

I picked up a pen and flipped the pages to a blank page.

30 June 2008

Dear Adult Naomi,

*Oh my dayz! You are, like, a serious tree hugger! I
have just read what you wrote at the beginning of the
diary and, well, it was kind of fascinating, even though
a bit Yoda's underpants!*

Still, I kind of get that with all of the continuously

*crappy things that have happened to you – well, to us –
that you had to do some soul searching, but please stop
with the self-help books! You've got* waaaayyy *too many
at home and I think you could write your own by now.
Anyway, in case you were wondering, I have brought you
to Egypt because I think you need a serious break and,
well, like L'Oréal says, 'You're worth it'! Hahahaha! And
the guy who brought our suitcases up is, like, TOTALLY
FIT!! Way better looking than Robert Harris, and I think
he's flirting with me! Oh, and I definitely think we are
meant to be here, because Phoenixes are, like, burned,
go through a death, and then they rise from the ashes
and live again and, well, I kind of reckon that's what
you're like – you keep getting back up, no matter how
many times you get knocked down. No matter how many
times you get burned. You keep coming back.*

 I hope you come back.

  Love,

   Teen Nay x

My eyes grew heavy as I thought of creation and the invisible energy that was responsible for vibrations, and as I drifted out of consciousness and into subconsciousness, my mind seemed to, like, stop for a second in the space in between. I wasn't fully asleep, but I wasn't awake either.

And that's when I saw it.

To the right of my bed on the wall was the biggest, longest, blackest scorpion I had ever seen. Well, I had never seen one, so had nothing to compare it to, but I could swear it was the size of a small cat. I stared at it, as it sat perfectly still, watching me. Then it leapt from the wall, flew across me, and landed on the other side of the room.

'WHAT THE F**K WAS THAT?' I screamed. I flicked on the light and sat up in bed. My heart was beating so loud and fast I could hear it hammering against my chest. I rubbed my eyes and stared at the wall. There was nothing there. *It must have been a dream*, I thought. But it had felt so real.

I was majorly scared. I lay down and pulled the covers up to my chin, watching the walls warily for its reappearance. I kept the light on, just in case.

In the morning, I woke up feeling like I hadn't really slept at all. This wasn't how I'd wanted to start off my holiday. By the time I got myself showered and dressed, I'd missed breakfast but I was in time for Marvellous Mark's induction and I listened as he outlined the excursions the holiday company offered. I couldn't seem to wake myself up fully from a kind of trance state. I kept thinking about the flying scorpion. It had seriously freaked me out.

I hadn't eaten since arriving the night before and it was a while before lunch, so I went to buy some chocolate. Coming out of the shop, I noticed an empty stool outside another, brightly coloured shop. The windows were filled with glass and golden brass smoking pipes of all colours, shapes and sizes. The top shelves were packed with the prettiest glass bottles I had ever seen. I walked in and was hit with a barrage of smells that slapped my sleeping mind awake in an instant. Several large sticks of incense were burning from a table at the back of the room; the rest of the scents came from rows and rows of bottles of perfume on glass shelves lining the dark blue and yellow silk-draped walls. Near the entrance of the shop at the left wall were two small sofas facing each other and a table scattered with magazines. I started to feel a little dizzy, so I sat down. A soft female voice was singing in the background and I looked up to see a small handheld CD player on the table. I watched the blue display, thinking how beautiful her voice sounded and how hypnotic the Arabic music was, when the old man I'd seen yesterday walked through a curtained door from the back of the shop, carrying a silver pot. I stood up quickly and, feeling my head rush, tried to fight the urge to flop back into the chair. I needed to get out of there.

'Tea?' asked the tiny old man. He had a kind voice.

I wasn't sure if I should drink the Egyptian water, but I really needed a drink at that moment so I nodded and watched him pour tea into a small glass. He sat on a stool next to the table and beckoned for me to sit on the other stool opposite him. I took the glass, said, '*Shukran*,' which I'd found out from Marvellous Mark was Egyptian for 'thank you', and sat down. As he poured himself a glass, I took a good look at him. He was dressed in dark trousers and a frayed, dark blue jumper with orange and yellow stains. The crumpled red collar of his shirt stuck out from the top of it. He seemed old, but his hair was jet black and thick with only a few grey hairs above his ears, which I noticed immediately because they were way too big for his small head. He had little black oval-shaped eyes that disappeared when he smiled and his deep laughter lines reminded me of small fans placed on the side of his face. He had a large nose, thin lips, and when he smiled, he revealed that several of his front teeth were missing; the rest were coffee- and tobacco-stained. His skin was a red-brown colour, weathered by so many years in the sun, and he had grey stubble across his jaw and underneath his chin.

Like an Egyptian Mr Miyagi, I thought.

I took a sip of the hot, sweet tea and it tasted really good, so I took another, larger sip.

'Mmm, good.'

He smiled and drank his with a loud slurping noise. He spoke to me in Arabic.

'Oh, I'm not Egyptian. I'm from the UK,' I laughed.

'Oh.' He chuckled. 'Engalish?'

'Yes.' I laughed again, not sure of the joke.

'Your first time in Egypt?' Laden with a thick, throaty Arabic accent, this man's English was impeccable.

'Yes, it is.' I sipped some more. The dizziness had gone and the tea was lifting my spirits.

'You are alone?'

I nodded. 'Yes, I came to Egypt all by myself.' I threw my shoulders back slightly and stuck out my chest, proud as a peacock. This made the old man laugh again. I shrank and sipped my tea. *What is so funny?*

'No husband?' he asked me, frowning.

'Totally not!' I replied, thinking of Adult Naomi's saddo diary entries about my two dads.

He shrugged his shoulders. 'You will be married,' he said matter-of-factly, as if he knew something I didn't.

And then he looked into my eyes intently. 'You deserve a good husband, good love for beautiful woman, yes?' The last

---

* *Mr Miyagi* – the cool Japanese dude who taught the actor Ralph Macchio how to fight in the 1984 film *The Karate Kid*.

word was a question and all of a sudden I felt like I wanted to cry. I didn't understand why what he had said wigged me out, so I took another sip of tea instead.

He smiled again. 'My name is Mo, Mohammed.'

'My name is Naomi.'

'Yoni?'

'Nay-omi.'

'Yomi,' he tried again.

Okay, so maybe his English wasn't as impeccable as I'd thought. I later realized that he wasn't actually trying to pronounce my name as he had heard it; he was trying to come up with words he knew that sounded similar, if not the same as Naomi.

I took out a pen and a piece of paper from my bag and wrote NA-OMI in big black letters. He repeated after me and said, 'Na (nah) Omi (homie),' and that's what he called me from then on. 'Nahomie', which, said quickly enough, sounded like he was saying 'Ma homie', which to me sounded like Tupac rapping poetic lyrics to his friend. I liked it and I decided not to correct him again.

When I finished my tea, I suddenly felt very calm. I yawned and threw my hand up to my mouth to hide my tiredness, not wanting him to take offence and think I was bored. He didn't; instead, he laughed his strange laugh, lit a filter-less cigarette, and offered me one. I refused politely.

'You are tired, Nahomie.'

I laughed and nodded.

'You like the perfumes?' He pointed to the intricately designed bottles on the walls.

'Yes.' I inhaled and braced myself for the sales pitch. Here we go. I should have seen it coming – the tea, the friendliness, the 'you need a good husband' spiel was all to soften me up so he could get me to part with my cash. Duh!

He reached his hand through the curtain and pulled out a blue glass bottle with a golden yellow stopper, opened it, and tipped red oil onto his nicotine-stained fingers. He rubbed it between his thumb and forefinger, testing the consistency, then gestured for me to hold out my hands palms up. I held them out and he poured two drops of oil on both wrists. He demonstrated with his own wrists that I should rub them together. The oil was one of the most gorgeous scents I had ever smelled. It was thick and sweet like treacle, mixed with the musky smell you get from damp wood after an autumn rain. I took another breath and could smell the new-born baby smell and the old-lady lavender and rose otto scent. A weird mix that somehow smelled great together. 'Oh, it's beautiful,' I exclaimed. It made me want to lie down, curl up with my nose next to my hands, and sleep.

'You go, you sleep, Nahomie,' Mo said.

'Yes, yes, I will and maybe no dreams of scorpions,' I mumbled to myself.

'Scorpions?' His eyes widened and his smile dropped.

'Erm . . . yes . . . Scor-pi-ons,' I said slowly and quietly.

He went very quiet and stared at me through squinted eyes. The silence was deafening; my heart started to drum to the same beat as the night before. I decided to explain.

'You see, what happened, right, was, like, I was really tired last night and I fell asleep, except I wasn't asleep, and then there was this, like, big, HUGE (I opened my arms to indicate the size of the beast) black, shiny scorpion on my wall and it flew across the room, across my body. And landed on the wall opposite.' I narrowed my eyes and whispered, 'And it was, like, watching me.'

'Yes?'

'Err, and then, well, I woke up and . . . erm . . . nothing.'

He seemed mesmerized by my words. He was silent for what felt like aeons while I stood nervously biting my lip, wondering why, and then he said just one word.

'Serket.'

'Sorry.'

'No sorry. Serket.'

I shook my head to show him I didn't understand.

'Serket,' he repeated.

I was majorly confused. 'Circuit?' I said. Maybe he was talking about racing cars, but what did this have to do with scorpions?

'Yes, Serrrrr-ket.'

Mo took the same pen and paper I had pulled out before and wrote on it the word 'SERKET'. I looked at it and then at him. Was I just supposed to keep repeating this word?

'Serrrrr-ket,' I tried.

'Yes! Serket. Queen of the Scor-pi-os, the Scorpion Queen.'

As soon as he said this, everything seemed to, like, lift completely and the trance-like state was gone. It was like when I had seen the phoenix the day before. The dying, the burning, the rising from the ashes, and starting again. Like the Phoenix. The Scorpion. Like me. I was supposed to be in the future.

'Serket,' I said out loud.

'Yes. The Scorpion Queen. She come from the darkness, the

night, into the light, the sun.' He put his hand to his chest and pointed the other hand to the sky and then down at me. 'She very powerful, very, very, very old. She sent to protect you, she will protect you.'

'Protect me?' I thought about the night I tried to kill myself. Protected – hadn't I heard that when I was praying I wouldn't die? And hadn't I heard it again when I read the diaries?

'Serket,' I repeated.

'Yes, she . . . she grab the throat . . . of your enemies.' He grabbed the air with his hand as if throttling an invisible neck. 'She heal the pain, the sting of your pain; she make you better.'

The pain, my pain, Adult Naomi's pain. I felt like I wanted to cry, but good tears, tears of relief.

'Protection,' he said.

The door opened and I turned around to see an old couple walk in. I turned back to Old Man Mo (my nickname for him) but he was messing around with the CD. I didn't know what else to do; what he had told me had left me speechless. Protection!

'Aaah, good afternoon. You like the perfumes?' His eyes lit up and he was addressing his new customers, like I had disappeared, so I picked up my bag quietly and said '*Shukran*' to him. He nodded without looking at me, and I made my way out of the shop. From the shop to my room, only one word swam inside my head: 'Serket'.

I fell into my bed listening to the waves, smelling the perfume on my wrists, and thinking of my visit the night before from Serket the Scorpion Queen.

I was exhausted but picked up the diary.

Dear Adult Naomi,

I think I got one of those universal messages you always write about. Okay, so I did get sent a big black scorpion the size of Steven Seagal's ponytail, but I met this weird old man from one of the shops today and I think I understood what he was saying. I kinda get it: like, no matter what you have been through – no, what we have been through – we have somehow been protected. I didn't get it at first but am thinking maybe it was this Serket. Old Man Mo said she is the Scorpion Queen and I think maybe that stopped things from getting all Silence of the Lambs *for you so you didn't end up locked in a padded jail cell, making weird noises with your tongue. Maybe me turning up isn't necessarily a bad thing, maybe I am helping Serket, maybe I am your protector, or maybe I am the Scorpion Queen and I have woken up in the future to sort your – no, our – life out. Heal the pain, heal the sting, heal your pain, my pain, and make it better.*

Yes, I think that's right; it feels right anyway.

I will try and make it better. In fact, I think things are already getting better.

Yeah!

Love,

Teen 'Scorpion Queen' Nay x

11

Teenage Dreams

*Woman cannot discover
new oceans
until she has courage
to lose sight of the shore.*

ANDRE GIDE

I spent the next eight days of my holiday in the company of
MEN!

After eating breakfast and being waited on hand and foot
by the waiters (all men), I would drink tea and have my daily
talk with Old Man Mo, discussing everything from Egyptian
politics to David Beckham. He never mentioned Serket again,
but it was okay. I got it.

I would call Simone and say hi to Leo and then sunbathe on
the beach until lunchtime, where I would be waited on hand
and foot by more men and write in the diary. I eventually gave
in to Adult Naomi's strange taste in music and, after listening
to her on the iPod, realized Kylie had dropped the Minogue
and had obviously become sexy since leaving Ramsay Street.

I found, much to my disgust, that as the days went past I was actually becoming a bit of a Kylie fan! I figured Adult Naomi had never really been open and free with her womanliness and she had spent way too much of her life in fear. So I deemed it my feminine responsibility to flash a big smile at any man I could and swing my hips in time to the Kylie theme tunes in my head, creating a kind of mental magnetism.

I snorkelled in the Red Sea amongst a pod of dolphins, alongside the underwater guide Muktarr, who held my hand and showed me his moves. I floated carelessly, brazenly watching his lithe, muscled chocolate-brown arms carry his toned body across the water, and was seriously impressed with his talent for making jungle animals out of towels.

I hung around with Bebo and his Marlboro-smoking boys, drinking Pepsis and laughing at the wack jokes he would tell. Bebo was the hotel's go-to guy when you wanted an excursion into the desert and the rest of the hotel's young workers seemed to look up to him. He spoke Italian, German, English and Arabic, and had learned all of his English from MTV. This guy's every second word was taken from a line from a rap or rock song. It was this strange mix of 'Yeah, Dude' and 'G UNIT' at the end of every sentence and some words had an almost Texan drawl while others could not disguise his thick Egyptian accent, so sounded like a strange Scottish-cockney hybrid. I called him and his gang the United Colours of Bebotton and he sang Enrique Iglesias songs and taught me Arabic swear words. I taught him how to do the running man dance and the MC Hammer 'swing your pants' one!

Through chilling with Bebo and his boys, I met Paulo and his quad bike. Paulo was tall, full of major muscles, and totally fit. His slicked-back hair and ponytail gave him this Italian sexiness, which was mental, because he was, like, Egyptian.

Before I knew it, I found myself on the back of Paulo's bike, speeding through the desert, arms wrapped around his rock-hard torso, screaming wildly and thinking of Serket.

And then there was Ali, a very intelligent, poised young man who took me on a beautiful horse called Warda through the desert to meet the Bedouin people, where I drank tea and tried a shisha pipe (bluuurgh). We talked about how badly the indigenous Bedouins were treated. He gave me a lecture on smoking and I quote, 'Really bad for you and you will die a slow and horrible death,' and this prompted me to write only one entry into the diary that night.

6 July 2008

Dear Adult Naomi,

A few points I must make for you for when you come back:

1. First, get rid of those friends! Not 'cause they are bad, they are just sooooo not like you and that's not, like, cool at all! (And listen to TLC's song 'What about your friends' if you forget.)

2. Second, quit smoking! 'Cause I am having a really hard time with this body! Your chest feels like it's wrapped in elastic bands.

3. When you get some sun, the spots and dark circles disappear, so, like, go on regular holidays!

4. Totally stop with the needy puppet-lookin' boyfriends! There's way too many totally fit gorge men out there,

who are, like, strong, sexy and really smart and, like, so
INTO YOU!

5. *You are confident, sexy, strong and smart and DON'T*
YOU FORGET IT!!

   Love from me!
      Teen 'Ooohh, on a TLC tip' Nay x

And last, but certainly not least, was Ahmed; romantic,
dreamy Ahmed, who I flirted with on a regs – well, every time
he came to clean my room. And who left me pretty arrangements on my bed made from flowers and swans constructed
out of white towels, leaving me to wonder if all Egyptian men
went to some sort of terry towel origami college?

I fluttered my eyelashes at Ahmed so much that he asked
me out on a date. I freaked out. Date? Me? I was only fifteen.
My dad would've killed me! But he didn't quite get this answer
and I mumbled something about a messy break-up and not
wanting to get him fired and scuttled sheepishly to the balcony until he had finished cleaning the room.

And it was while I sat looking out at the sea that I thought
how sad it was that Adult Naomi had only ever felt safe with
men who reminded her of my dad. Life wasn't supposed to
be like that. You were supposed to feel safe around any man,
all different types of men, and not feel threatened, not feel
like at any moment your trust would be abused. I needed to
believe different. I wanted to experience different. The world,
my world, couldn't be this damaged.

So I took a deep breath, went back into the room and told
Ahmed to pick me up when he had finished his shift.

*

Ahmed came at nine o'clock. I opened the door to find him
smiling shyly and holding a bunch of flowers. Out of his uniform, he looked even more majorly fit. He was wearing black
jeans, white trainers, and a bright white T-shirt, which made
his caramel skin look even more delicious and his dark eyes
sparkle. I took the flowers and my face went all spazoidy red
hot. To this, he gave a nervous laugh and I could have sworn
his teeth were whiter than his T-shirt.

I closed my door and he held on to my hand and led me
down the stairs and across the hotel complex. I prayed my
hands wouldn't go all sweaty as I tried to walk in step with
him. He walked confidently, like he was proud to be by my
side. I wore a cerise-pink cotton dress with thin straps and a
pair of gold sandals and carried a small white cardigan over
my arm. I had bought the dress before the holiday, reckoning
Adult Naomi needed not to be afraid of wearing the colour
pink anymore.

'I am happy you are here with me,' he proclaimed, and
stared at me intensely.

'Me too.' My stomach gave a nervous tickle and I hung my
head down in slight embarrassment, thinking, *Oh my God,
what is going on? Get it together, Nay.*

We walked together for what seemed like ages, through the
hotel and past the shops. I started to get more anxious and
asked where exactly he was taking me.

'Oh, this is where we stay, the staff from the hotel. We have
our own place.' He pointed to a large white apartment building situated outside of the gates away from the hotel. It had
a couple of smaller buildings next to it and was surrounded
by desert.

Oh no, oh no! I thought. *Quick, run, get out of here. He's a serial killer. He's going to kidnap you and kill you or sell you to the highest bidder.*

I called on Serket instead of giving in to my paranoid thoughts.

Ahmed stopped and held my gaze. It was so freaking me out; I wanted to look away, but I was spellbound by his gorgeousness.

'Naomi, you are safe with me; I will not let you come to any harm.' He frowned. 'I want to take you for food, look,' he said, pointing at the smaller buildings. 'There is a restaurant for us, we eat, we drink, we have a good time. But I can take you back to the hotel if you are not comfortable with me.'

The question stopped the serial killer thoughts in their tracks. I didn't wanna leave him.

'No.' I looked down at his hand, holding firmly on to mine. I didn't know why, but I felt okay. 'I want to go with you, Ahmed.'

His face lit up and he led me to a small, softly lit cafe-type restaurant, picking a table in a quiet corner. Apart from one waiter, who I think was the cook and the owner, the place was empty. Our table was the only one covered with a white tablecloth; it had a small glass jar with a single pink flower on it. Ahmed pulled my chair out for me. I sat down and he sat opposite, smiling. The waiter came over with a large green jar, lit the candle inside of it, and placed it on the table. He looked at Ahmed, eyebrows raised, and nodded his head in approval. Ahmed smiled shyly. This made me relax and the waiter handed us some menus.

'We have good food here, not the hotel food. This is real Egyptian food,' he said, with pride.

I looked down at the menu. It was in Arabic. We both burst out laughing.

'I will order for you, if you please.'

'Yes, I please.' I grinned moronically.

'You are very beautiful, Naomi,' he said softly. His face grew serious and I grew sloppy, my stomach flipping upside down.

'Very beautiful,' he echoed to himself.

Whoa! My first proper date!

Ahmed ordered us a dish he called *torly* which had lamb and vegetables in it, and was eaten with bread and rice. It was bloody hard to look kriss while eating the food with my hands. The waiter gave us knives and forks, but it felt right to eat this way, so I copied Ahmed, trying my best not to get sauce around my mouth or *molokhia* leaves in my teeth.

Ahmed still somehow managed to look beautiful while eating his and telling me about his life. He was the eldest of nine children, he said proudly, showing me a picture on his phone of his mother, who didn't look old enough to be his mum, let alone have nine children. He then showed me a picture of his youngest brother who was, like, two years of age. It made me think of JJ and I wondered what he was like when he was two. I wished I could remember, but some memories were still missing. Nonetheless, I told Ahmed about him and about Leo and Simone and Art. He asked about my mum, but I just shrugged my shoulders and said she lived in London. He looked a little embarrassed, but changed the subject, telling me he studied engineering in Cairo, but worked in

Marsa during the summer break. He asked me about my time in Egypt and what I did for a living.

Crap, I thought. *I am sooooo unemployed.*

'I, erm . . . I am t . . . t . . . taking some time out to f . . . f . . . finish my psychology degree,' I stuttered.

'Aaah, the mysteries of the mind?' He laughed, his eyes twinkling. 'This I am very interested in. I have a friend who is studying the same at university. What have you learned about the human mind? My friend, he talks a lot about it; I am interested to know your opinion.' He clasped his hands together and leaned forward.

Beads of sweat started to trickle down the sides of my face and my heart started to beat fast. One, because he was asking me an intellectual boffin-type question and two, because his total hotness was too close to me.

I avoided his gaze and looked up at the wall at all of the pictures of the pyramids, the citadel and the gold Arabic writing. I thought of waking up in the future and reading Adult Naomi's writings in her diaries. Then I thought of me carrying on her future and writing it to her. It suddenly popped into my head and I got it. I turned to Ahmed and stared into his coffee-brown eyes.

'You have to get it out.' I looked back up at the gold Arabic writing. 'No matter how hard it is, no matter what it is, you have to get it out. You can't keep everything locked up inside of your head. Do you know what I mean?' Was I making sense?

He nodded, intrigued, and leaned forward a little more, making me feel faint.

I continued. 'Erm, I mean, the mind, it's precious . . . like, it's a part of you, you need it. It needs you and you must take care of it like you would, say, your heart? You know?'

He nodded again; a smile curled at the corner of his mouth. I wanted to drop out of my chair right there and then. 'Erm, and yeah.' I composed myself. 'So, I think, you need to get it all out, because if you don't, it breaks.'

'The mind?' He looked concerned.

'Yeah, and, well, the only way to fix it is if you get out what broke it in the first place.'

He leaned back and gave me a relaxed smile, his eyes full of admiration. I smiled back and gave myself a mental fist pump. I made sense; it made sense.

'You are a very smart woman, Naomi. A very beautiful, special, and smart woman,' he said intensely, as if all of a sudden I needed to know what he was thinking seriously and quite urgently.

I grabbed hold of the side of my chair, the feeling in my legs gone completely. My face flushed red and I felt hot; my mouth went dry and my palms began to sweat. I was a total wreck. I was *sooooo* not acting like a thirty-two-year-old.

I gave a small nervous and giggly smile. He laughed and turned to the waiter to order some sweets. I took a sip of my water, trying to figure out what had just happened to me, and realized I hadn't noticed that the restaurant had slowly filled with staff from the hotel, who were sitting at the tables, sharing food. I felt shy and a little awkward, so I put on my cardigan.

Ahmed noticed and put his hand on mine. 'You are okay here,' he reassured me.

And then the door burst open and the United Colours of

Bebotton spilled in. They spoke loudly, shouting and laughing to the owner. Bebo started singing as he pulled tables together for him and his gang.

'Hey, my sister!' he shouted over. 'Wassssupppp?'

I laughed and instantly relaxed. He gave a knowing nod to Ahmed, then went back to his loud argument with his boys. Even though he spoke Egyptian Arabic, I could make out the words 'Slim' and 'Shady' and 'white rappers'. I had no clue who he was talking about, but was sure it wasn't Vanilla Ice.

It got really loud and busy in the restaurant so we got up to leave. Ahmed paid the bill. We said our goodbyes and thanked the owner and I followed Ahmed into the warm desert air. He took a hold of my hand and we walked slowly back to the hotel.

I was just thinking I'd had such a good night and that I didn't want to leave him, when he said, 'I had a really good night. I do not want to leave you,' and squeezed my hand gently. 'The beach is quiet. We could sit down there?' He looked at me hopefully. I nodded, wigged out at his mind-reading skills.

There was a circular wooden drinks bar in the middle of the beach. Ahmed jumped over the counter and grabbed some hotel towels from underneath the bar. He laid them down on the sand near a large tree trunk and beckoned for me to sit, so I took off my sandals and cardigan and sat down. He sat and leaned up against the trunk. Wanting to feel his arms around me, I shuffled up towards him. He did the mind-reading thing again, wrapping his arms around me and pulling me closer, where I rested my head on his chest, feeling really chilled. We both watched the dark water lap against the beach.

'Thank you, Ahmed. I have had a lovely night.'

'You are welcome, Naomi. I am happy you are here with me,' he whispered.

'Me too.' I nestled further into his arms and closed my eyes. I listened to the gentle rushing sound of the waves; it sounded like music. Like a lullaby. So much so that I felt calm, relaxed, and sleepy. I gave a small smile when I realized for the first time in a long time I felt safe.

My holiday was almost over but not before I got to take a trip to the Great Pyramids of Giza. On the plane, I sat next to two sisters who were staying at the same hotel. Toni was the elder. At nineteen, she was slim and freckled with short blonde hair, reserved and nowhere near as open as her younger sister. Ashley was seventeen, and reminded me of a human version of an Ice Cream Doll, with long blonde hair, a button nose and freckled cheeks. She had a curious expression and bright blue eyes. We chatted for a while and then settled back for the short flight to Cairo.

I thought about my first ever real date the night before. Ahmed had been a total gentleman. We'd sat on the beach, talking until the sun came up, and then he had walked me back to my room. I'd got all tongue-tied when he told me over and over how beautiful I was and how much he had enjoyed my company, and when he kissed me softly on the lips, I almost dropped on the bedrock floor there and then.

All the attention I had received over the time I had been in Egypt made me feel well righteous and *sooooo* kriss. I felt, like, this pride in myself I had never felt before, a bonfire of my own vanity (Mrs Doughtily had made us read Tom Wolfe for English lit.). I couldn't help but marvel at the way the heat of my new-found sexiness had elicited so much attention from all of these gorgeous men.

It was short-lived. Any fake confidence I had amassed during my flirtatious stay at Marsa Alam soon came to an abrupt end.

In Cairo, a driver met us at the airport and led us to our spacious air-conditioned coach. When we were seated, a short young man hopped up the steps enthusiastically and greeted us with a big smile, a whoop, and a loud 'good morning'. He wore a checked shirt, faded jeans and silver-rimmed glasses with thick lenses that sat on his broad nose and moved up and down every time he spoke. He informed us that he was a student at the University of Cairo, a proud Muslim man who was honoured to be our guide through the city this very day, and that his name was 'Smile'. I gave a squeal of delight at his name and his infectious jovialness and waited for him to squeal back. He didn't. Instead he squinted at me through his glasses, frowned, and carried on with his 'welcome to Cairo' speech. I thought maybe he had been mistaken and didn't mean to look at me that way.

For some reason, from that moment on, Smile did everything in his power to make sure I knew he didn't particularly care for me by giving me so many dirty looks I was surprised someone didn't offer me a bar of soap. By the time we were sitting in the Citadel Mosque, I made sure I sat as far away as possible from him. I eventually wandered from the crowd to avoid his disapproving stares.

I had also somehow got on the wrong side of the women standing at the entrance to the mosque, who gave me the filthiest looks and practically threw a large green covering over me to hide my bare arms and legs.

I was beginning to guess that maybe covering my head in a white wrap to match my sleeveless low-cut dress had not been such a good idea. There was a method to my offensive madness. I had always adored the sun, but ever since I was a child, I found if I spent too long under its rays I would end up with terrible headaches. It became wise for me to stay in the shade as much as possible or, even better, cover my head. Unfortunately, this meant that I grew sensitive to the UV rays and burned easily, the top of my head included. When I'd been trying to jog my memory, I had looked at many photographs. Judging by the ones of Adult Naomi wearing wide-brimmed hats and carrying parasols, I had reached the conclusion that this problem had got worse, not better. I was adamant that my day spent in Cairo under the hot Egyptian sun was not going to end with a burnt scalp, shoulders and nose, so I had packed plenty of sunscreen, wrapped my hair in a beautiful white cotton cloth, and was carrying my pink parasol.

Maybe it was the parasol that irked Smile, or the wrapped hair and my audacity at showing my legs and arms that pissed the women off. Whatever it was, I realized by the time we left the mosque that I wasn't going to find Cairo as friendly as Marsa Alam. In fact, I was met with downright hostility and Smile seemed to revel in it. When we reached the famous Egyptian Museum, I quickly got myself lost and made sure I stayed far away from him. This further infuriated him; as far as he was concerned, I should have followed his tour of the museum, and listened intently like the rest of the group to what he had to say.

I gave him my best I-am-fifteen-and-you-can't-tell-me-what-to-do look and walked away from him. I was hot, bothered, thirsty, and frankly pissed off with the amount of dirty looks I was getting from the people of Cairo! I refused to take my wrap off and instead went straight to the exhibitions I wanted to see. When I had finished, I bought a can of Pepsi and sat outside the museum with an obese family from Doncaster who said the word 'fuck' at the beginning, in the middle and at the end of every sentence. They reminded me of Manchester and, for a small moment, I had a longing to be back under the grey skies of home, learning how to speak without pronouncing my Ts.

As I was thinking that maybe Manchester was starting to feel like home, it suddenly hit me why Naomi had brought a child into this world: she needed family. She needed to belong and know unconditional love when everything around her seemed so conditional. She needed a home and that home was where her heart was. Leo and Simone were her home. And it didn't matter whether that was in a big house with a pool and cars or a small house with a broken gate and a strange cat. As long as there was love there, as long as she belonged and felt safe there, that was all that mattered.

As Smile came out of the museum, it was clear he had had enough of my solo rebellion. He was obviously angry that I had left the group and told me in no uncertain terms that it was in my best interest to stick with him. 'Cairo is a dangerous place and bad things will happen to you.'

I laughed, flipped my parasol up, and walked away from him. He followed.

'You are very rude,' he called after me.

'No, YOU are very rude.' I raised my voice, and people stopped and stared.

'But you have not followed the group, you do not listen, you have no respect.'

'I don't have to follow the group. Why should I have to listen to you? And respect is earned.' As hard as I felt, I wanted to burst into tears and I very much wanted this man to leave me alone.

The group were trickling out of the museum and coming over to us. The pink parasol wasn't providing me with enough shade so I moved from him and sat on a wall under the cooler shade of a large tree.

'Listen to me, I will get into trouble if I lose you.'

'I am a fifteen . . . no, thirty-two-year-old woman.' I stood up and he took a step back in surprise. 'I can take care of myself and you will not lose me. I am not a child.' Tears were welling up in my eyes. What was this man's problem with me?

Ashley came and stood next to me. 'Are you okay?' she asked.

'No, I'm not,' I replied. Turning back to Smile, I said, 'I don't understand what it is I have done to you exactly, but I would prefer it if you just left me alone and didn't speak to me for the rest of the day and I won't speak to you.' By this point, Smile had begun to look embarrassed and slightly sorry.

'Come on.' Ashley took me by the arm and led me to the gated exit. Toni followed.

We walked back to the coach where Toni asked the driver if he could switch the air conditioning on. The cool air helped me swallow back my hot tears. I was furious. Who the hell did this man think he was? I asked the girls.

'He's acting like my dad.' I turned to Ashley. 'I mean, what the smeg?'

'What does smeg mean?' she asked in wide-eyed innocence.

It was at that moment that I felt truly alone. As great as my holiday had been so far, I couldn't escape the fact that I was still fifteen and still in the future, where *Red Dwarf* was a 'classic' and I was stuck in a place where antiquated ideas about women still existed. It was the complete opposite to the future world I had woken up into and the way the men at the hotel treated me. In my confusion, I burst into tears. Ashley put her arm around me and cursed Smile with as many cockney expletives as she could come up with; half of them I didn't understand but they made me laugh and I felt better for it because she was on my side.

'He's coming back.' Toni, who had been quiet up until then, gave me an encouraging smile. I wiped my swollen eyes, took a swig of warm water, and put my large sunglasses on. I was not going to give him the satisfaction of seeing me upset.

Everyone clambered onto the coach and I could feel their eyes staring at me, wondering if I was going to start something with their beloved tour guide. But I kept my face towards the window and didn't look around until I woke up half an hour later outside of the Pyramids of Giza.

Smile wouldn't let us off the coach until he had given his version of who he reckoned had built the pyramids. He mocked the theory that aliens may have built them and at this point I didn't care anymore; as far as I was concerned my mum said that they were built by aliens and Smile was wrong so I scoffed at him like the naughty schoolgirl at the back of the class.

'You have fifteen minutes, and then the coach will leave for the Nile.'

'*Fifteen minutes?*' I couldn't take any more. The cherry on the top of the whole unpalatable cake of Smile's attitude was getting to spend time inside the great pyramids of Giza and now this man was telling me I would have to run around the monuments under the hot sun and could forget about actually going inside.

'Yes, there is not much time and people have asked to go on the Nile.'

'Well, then those people need to pay for an excursion that takes them on the Nile. I have waited all day for this and have paid *my* money for you to tell me that I am going to get fifteen minutes?'

'Please, please, the journey took longer than I anticipated.'

'That's because we spent nearly two bloody hours in your precious mosque!' I shouted at him.

I heard gasps from the back of the coach. I was bordering on serious political incorrectness and about to free-fall into anti-Islamic territory – well, to some anyway; to me, I was just majorly pissed off that I was only getting fifteen minutes to see one of the greatest wonders of the world.

This was personal. It was the last straw. I suddenly realized that to him and to everyone else, I really was a grown woman and I could tell him what I thought of him. 'You are rude, ignorant, and clearly think that sucking up to these people will get you far in life.' I waved my hand at the rest of the coach and gave them a dirty look for not being on my side.

Smile was speechless; I grabbed my bag and stormed off the coach, furious. I turned by the door and looked him straight in the eye. 'And I am putting in a complaint about you.' He looked horrified. I snapped my pink parasol in the air and flounced off.

In a show of solidarity, Ashley and Toni stuck their noses up at him and followed me towards the pyramids.

'He is a complete wanker and needs to jog on,' Toni remarked.

'Yeah, knob jockey. I don't wanna see the bloody Nile either,' Ashley agreed.

I shook my head at them both, too upset to speak. I just wanted to use what little time I had to see as much of the pyramids as possible. This meant walking around the largest one once and having pictures taken of me smiling, sitting on the large blocks of white stone under my parasol. I really wanted to burst into tears, but this time my womanly pride or my stubborn teenage dignity would not give him the satisfaction of seeing me upset.

As promised, the coach pulled away from the Pyramids fifteen minutes after we had arrived. I had given up being angry at Smile and what he thought about me. It didn't matter. Besides, the fear on his face the moment I had threatened to report him was mega and had made me feel so much better. I had taken back the power and a satisfied smugness hit me the same time as the realization that I was in Giza. This was when I felt that I shouldn't give it any more energy and needed to take in the beautiful surroundings. So I stood instead and marvelled at the Sphinx, an unbelievable feat of design and architecture. It was majestic and its mere presence sought to remind me that I had accomplished my goal: to bring Adult

Naomi to this marvellous ancient wonder and, even if it was just for a brief moment in time, allow me to absorb all of its gloriousness. If only for her.

When we stopped at a petrol station, Smile approached me. 'My friend, my friend.' He edged tentatively to my table.

'Oh, I am your friend now?' I said incredulously.

'I think maybe you and I . . . we . . . how do you say? Got in the wrong foot.' He shifted from one foot to the other.

I couldn't help myself. 'It's *off* on the wrong foot and I have no clue what you mean.' I stared at him, wide-eyed and innocent.

Visibly uncomfortable with the whole situation, he started to sweat. 'I say we do not need this to be so disagreeable with each other. I am just trying to do a good job.'

At the mention of his job, his face grew worried and I realized at that moment that he really was afraid of losing it and I held all the employment cards. As wickedly divine as it felt, playing the villain didn't come naturally to me. I felt sorry for the poor div. I decided it was time to be honest with him.

'I don't understand what it was I did to you to make you not like me. From the moment I sat down on the coach, you were horrible to me, and then, to make matters worse, you ignored me, gave me horrible filthy looks all day and then demanded I follow you when I didn't even want to be around you.'

He shrugged his shoulders and hung his head in shame.

'I get it,' I continued. 'You are a Muslim man; you are proud of your Arabic ancestors and what they have done for Egypt. Yeah, I get it, but I am African and Egypt was North Africa before it was Arabia, and my ancestors built the pyramids, and they lied to us in school and made us watch films with Elizabeth Taylor in them, and . . .' I was going off topic; he looked confused. 'And I paid a lot of money to come here from England and fly to Cairo all the way from Marsa Alam' – he nodded his head like a chastised pupil – 'only to go on a tour of your history, not mine,' I finished.

He lifted his head up. 'Yes, I understand. I am sorry.'

I shrugged my shoulders. It was too little too late. The day was over; we were heading home and this man was apologizing because I had threatened his job. As sincerely as he said it, it felt insincere. Still, I nodded my head. 'Well, at least you listened, if nothing else.' I got up and walked back to the coach, and while it took us to the Nile I tried not to think about how my visit to Cairo had not turned out at all the way I had expected.

Back at my hotel room Ahmed had left his usual flower arrangement, but this time he had spelt LEO and NAOMI in an arch across the bed. I fell onto the flowers and burst into tears. I missed Leo; I missed Simone and Katie and Dean. It was time to go home. I didn't want to be on my own anymore and I knew I needed to leave. That night, out of sheer exhaustion, I slipped easily into a dreamless sleep.

I woke up feeling much better and determined not to spend my last day in Egypt in my room, so I dressed quickly, threw my bag on my shoulder, and made my way to the beach. I spotted an empty space close to the grand wall of rocks situated at the far end of the beach. The massive red-orange rock face provided the seclusion I craved, my very own private beach. I lay down on my towel, the hot sand sending waves of massaging heat kneading every tired knot from my body. It made me relax immediately.

When I thought about the day before, I realized Smile was ignorant; he had been judgemental and arrogant because he didn't know how to deal with me. So instead of giving me a chance and trying to get to know me, to understand me, he had tried to control me. Which felt kinda familiar. I realized that this had been happening to me since I was little. People trying to force me to be someone I am not. Force themselves on me.

Had Adult Naomi become so afraid of this that she had tried to bend and break herself to appease people? If you always think every time you're your 'real' self that you're gonna be attacked, then eventually, it is safer to be someone else. But this wasn't working anymore. I knew that this was what had caused the splits in her mind. In my mind.

Was this also true for my mum? All of the things she had said, the questions she had asked me that day I tried to kill myself. Were they really about me? Maybe they were questions she was asking herself. Maybe she was afraid because she had no answers for her own life. She couldn't figure out her point, her purpose.

Well, maybe being my true self means I have to stand alone, I thought. *There is a point to me, I have a purpose and just because I haven't figured it out yet, just because other people think they know me better than I do, and try to stop me or control what I say or do, then it doesn't mean I won't figure it out.*

I decided to write one more diary entry so I pulled Adult Naomi's diary out of my bag, grabbed a pen and began to write.

Dear Adult Naomi,

I think I know what happened to you – to us. I think we got lost, somewhere along the way, somewhere in the splits; who we really are – who you really are – got lost. And every now and then, we met a complete smeg (last time I use it, I promise) face, tosspotting wanker who thought it was okay to barf their own mentalist issues and their own complete wackness all over you. And we forgot, forgot somehow that most of that barf wasn't ours! We took it on, took it all on, and because it was heavy and he was not our brother (remember the song?) we got buried underneath all that spew like it was our responsibility. I think the books we read and the plays we were in taught us how to kind of split into all these different acting parts, so we could get through life, you know? Get through the crap. But you know what I have realized today is that I am me, you are you, we are we; it's me, Naomi, and I don't have to be what people want me to be. I'm okay, you are okay being yourself, and you need to start letting it all out, ALL of you out, every single bit, and well, if they don't like it, tell them to take a long running jump off a very short pier. Stop giving yourself total crapness for other people's ignorant, foolish idiocies. Speak your truth, be who you are, your true self, and don't apologize for it! I mean it, no matter who it makes feel uncomfortable or who doesn't like it. If it's yours, then it's you and no one can take that away from you. You know I'm glad I have come here and in case you don't remember any of this when you come back, I want you to know what I have realized on this holiday about life.

I realize it's not about people and what they think of me; it's about what I know about myself and who I really am, and in the end that's all that really matters.

Love from me,

Totally frickin' kriss biscuits Teen Nay xxx

I put the book down, closed my eyes and fell asleep on the beach, thinking about the future.

Sometime later, I opened my eyes and blinked at the blurred blue sky above me.

It felt like I had had one of the best, deepest sleeps I had ever had. I looked around and knew instantly that I, Adult Naomi, had returned to my body.

12

All About Eve

Everything has its time;
you can't force something
to happen
before it's meant to.
That's a true law,
a universal law.

Y. J.

The last thing I remembered was falling asleep crying, thinking about 'French Dude' and how much of a failure at life I was. Now two months had passed and I was back to seeing my life and my world from my perspective, but the odd thing was, I was carrying Teen Nay's memories of what had happened to her from those strange few weeks.

I knew that her whole experience of waking up in my future had brought her to one conclusion: that if life hadn't turned out the way she had expected, I was the only one responsible for changing it. Things that had happened to me in the past were out of my control. But as I held the fresh memories from her experience of my adult life, I realized the only true power I had lay in how I reacted to those experiences. She had set me free to do what I needed to do, to make sure that things stayed as normal as possible for Leo, but at the same time changed for me. Teen Nay had done it for us; now I needed to do it for us. I knew undoubtedly that I, Adult Naomi, had to change things.

I arrived back from the holiday refreshed, tanned and full of stories of Teen Nay's adventures, and as soon as I walked through the door Simone burst into tears.

'Oh my God.' She clasped her hands over her mouth.

'What?' I looked behind, thinking the taxi driver had followed me in.

'You, it's you!' She walked towards me and stood staring.

'Can you tell?'

'Straight away.' She gave me one of her back-breaking hugs and I relaxed into her arms. 'You're back, I've got my sister back.'

'I was always your sister,' I said to her, tears welling in my eyes.

She stepped back and laughed. 'I know, but seriously, how much "smeg for brains" can a woman take?'

We both stood crying and laughing and hugging each other.

'Oh my God, Sim, what a trip.'

'Egypt or the amnesia?'

'Both.' I paused. 'And, *chica*, thank you so much for everything, for keeping me sane, looking after Leo and . . . just everything.' I started to cry again.

She hugged me again. 'It's okay. I've always told you, if I can support you and Leo in any way, then I always will.'

I felt so grateful that throughout everything my sister had remained her calm and stoic self, trusted me to work through it and at the same time kept me out of the psychiatric ward.

Leo was happy to see me and I had missed him so much. He had changed a lot in two months and I was grateful that somehow Simone and Katie had managed to keep him protected from the whole amnesia experience. When I told him what had happened later on, he was surprised and then said, 'I wondered why you asked me what time I went to bed.' Then he laughed and carried on skateboarding.

It had been fascinating seeing the world from Teen Nay's perspective but now I was back, recycling, coffee shops, bizarre fashion and inflation were as normal to me as they had always been. I still remembered how to drive and use a mobile phone. And my slush puppy love for Leo was as strong if not stronger.

Their support and understanding gave me what I needed to sit down one night and read the diary entries Teen Nay had written for me. I saw that she wrote that I had extreme difficulty in using the word 'no'. I said yes even when I didn't want to do things and if I did feel brave enough to say no, I would feel guilt on a crazy level and at some point fall off that level into a large sea of shame and want to hide deep at the bottom of the ocean of my unworthiness. (*Dramatic*, she said. *I know*, I replied, *but sadly, true.*)

According to her, it seemed saying yes way too many times had caused all the problems in the first place and under no circumstances was she going to allow me to repeat the same mistakes again. This resulted in her writing about *Grange Hill*'s Zammo curled up in a corner, doped up on heroin, and the rest of the fifth-year kids rapping 'JUST SAY NO'. Teen

Nay felt I needed this reminder as clearly it hadn't penetrated my subconscious well enough the first time round.

Still, her Egypt experience had shown me what life could be like, if I could just let go of the constant fear. Let go of feeling threatened. She had shown me that it was okay to trust myself and that somehow, through it all, I was protected. I didn't quite fully understand that yet, but I knew I needed to find a way to trust her and thought about what Old Man Mo had said to her before she left. He shed a little tear when she said goodbye to him with hugs and thank yous, and gave her a bottle of Egyptian musk, saying to her 'Serket will always be with you.'

So, unlike me, Teen Nay had not disappeared. She still existed in my mind – in fact, she was resident in the 'house' – and she was watching what I would do next with a careful eye. I had no explanation as to why she hadn't left like I had but as I wondered how I was going to find a way through this situation and, above all, how I could make sure this never happened again, I found that my conversations with Teen Nay were happening daily. Perhaps because no one else could give me any answers, I turned to her for advice rather than the other people in my life. Every time something happened I would check in with her, and in a sort of inner dialogue I'd hear her voice giving me her often brutal fifteen-year-old opinion on all things Adult Naomi.

But it wasn't until one sunny July morning, whilst I lay on my bed staring at my beautifully decorated bedroom in awe of her and the force of change she had brought to my life, that I decided to close my eyes, breathe deeply and really focus on entering the 'house of my mind'.

It was easier than I'd anticipated; I was so relaxed and could clearly see the vision of Teen Nay lounging on her own bed in a beautiful bedroom on the first floor (very reflective of the beautiful bedroom she had given me in real life). I could see myself sitting on the edge of her bed and we both smiled at each other. She was young, beautiful and vibrant. Expectant energy seemed to emanate from her. All of a sudden she somehow managed to propel my mind back to a time when it all started. She wanted me to remember something important. We went back to when I was five.

Her: *Remember when Mum . . . I mean, Eve, had moved us into a squat?*

Me: *Yeah, I think so. Orange-brick house, on that quiet estate, the one with the Chinese neighbours? Didn't Aunty June accuse them of kidnapping Blacky the dog and eating it?*

Her: *Errrr . . . off topic! Anyway, remember the wall?*

Me: *The wall, the wall . . . erm . . . no, I don't . . . hang on, you mean . . . ? Oh yeah! You mean that night me and Simone took two small pencil stubs? I don't know whose idea it was . . .*

Her: *It was yours.*

Me: *Yeah, I remember now. I decided to use the light from the hallway to draw all over the wall next to our bed . . . yeah, I drew houses and a large park in great detail with swings and slides. I drew a post office, a bank, a bakery, and a green grocer's. Didn't I even add people to my small town, and then . . . didn't I put a forest next to it? With trees and woodland creatures and jungle animals?*

Her: *You so did!*

Me: *We drew all night until we couldn't keep our eyes open. I was buzzing that I had found a way to fall asleep living in the world I had just created, being able to do and say and go anywhere I wanted! But the next day, you know, Eve went ballistic.*

Her: *Majorly ballistic! Remember, she grounded you? And gave you a bucket of warm, soapy water and a wire scrubbing brush. You had to scrub off every single drawing.*

Me: *Yeah, I remember now. Gosh, I was devastated. We had both spent hours drawing these imaginary worlds full of amazing places and special people, and then we had to destroy them.*

Her: *Yeah, it was mega sad. You both started to cry.*

Me: *Yeah, but seeing the tears in my sister's eyes, I don't know . . . I remembered how happy my stories made her. I felt it was my responsibility to make her sadness go away.*

Her: *So you grabbed a pair of knickers.*

Me: *KNICKERS?!*

Her: *Yeah, remember, out of the bin bags our clothes were in? You put them on your head, stuck a pencil in your mouth, pretended it was a Woodbine and became—*

Me: *Edna Jacobs! The washerwoman who told stories!*

Her: *Finally!*

Me: *I remember. It made Simone laugh and I carried on telling her the stories we'd created even if we couldn't see them. You know, even though we had to scrub everything off the wall, it didn't matter because they carried on having great adventures. Yeah, because I knew I was Edna Jacobs, 'The Washer Woman Storyteller', and I was going to tell their stories.*

Her: *Yeah, Sim was well happy and you both stopped crying.*

Me: *I think I promised myself that I was going to have the same adventures as my characters and tell their tales to those that wanted to know, just to see their smile, and wipe away the tears.*

Her: *Totally.*

Me: *But clearly, this was a psychological reaction to the distress of being uprooted and taken from the only life I had known. Eve running away from Liverpool wasn't because of the riots; it was because she was hiding from a domestically violent environment, so this meant that my memories of the childhood I'd had so far were fading. And clearly I had no choice but to embrace my new life of squat-dwelling storyteller.*

Her: *Ugh! Psycho bibble babble!! Who cares?*

Me: *But I was five.*

Her: *Duh, yeah! And you already knew what you wanted to be then! What you wanted to do with your life. You just forgot!*

(I mentally saw myself crawl up to the top of the bed; she shuffled over and I lay down next to her. We both lay there, staring up at the ceiling of the house of my mind.)

Her: *Remember Joseph and his video camera? All of the plays and musicals and singing we did for him?*

Me: *I always wanted to control the stage production.*

Her: *You mean you wanted to boss everyone around!*

Me: *Ha-ha-ha! Yeah!*

Her: *Remember after that you wanted to be an actress and would sit in front of the mirror smoking a pen, pretending it* was a Benson and Hedges, pretending you were some drug-crazed criminal being interviewed by an officer from The Bill. *Erm, dude!* Took the drug-crazed bit slightly too far.

Me: *Yeah, but my soliloquy on being a reluctant grass and informing on my 'well hard' gangster boyfriend was to die for. It had tears and everything.*

Her: *We were good at English language and literature, weren't we? It was our favourite subject in school. I knew I wanted to be a journalist when Miss Doughtily gave me an A for my teabag-stained Veronian newspaper and my wicked article on the scandal of Romeo and Juliet shagging each other.*

Me: *Gosh, yeah! I wanted more William and I understood Chaucer, I really did; that love in heaven and pain in hell thing, I got it. Remember Mr Marsham, the English lit. teacher?*

Her: *And his coloured bow ties that always matched his glasses, and his striped shirts?* (In mocking posh voice) *I have a fervent passion for all works Ye Olde English.*

Me: *Ha-ha-ha! I felt like he was my mythical Timmy Mallet, except large volumes of text were his Thor-like weapon and the resulting feelings after reading were my solatium. I lapped up any book he would put in front of me, and everyone else would bitch and moan. But I would give a squeal of delight at the sheer volume of the works, and, nervously biting my lip, enquire as to how long we had to scale the prodigious literary mountain.*

Her: *Oh my dayz! Stop, woman! You've got the message! We like words. We like to write! So WRITE!*

So, eventually accepting that I didn't need to come up with a million and one reasons to write, and spurred on by mine and Teen Nay's conversation about my mind and our memories, I started to write short stories based on my mega mental experiences. I swapped the self-empowerment class for a creative writing one. This got me out of the house and around people who wanted to share their own stories.

It was only after I read out my first funny piece, titled *Battle of the Bacofoil* (it was about being angry because I had burnt my Christmas turkey), and received a round of applause afterwards, that I really started to take what Teen Nay had said seriously.

Katie and Simone read my short stories and loved them, and after another day sitting in my room, staring at the Hollywood walls in awe of Teen Nay, I meditated and entered the 'house' to find her in the bedroom, sitting at a desk, holding a pen.

Her: *So you like your bedroom, then?*
Me: *Very much.*
Her: *And the colour – it's sick, right?*
Me: *Sick?*
Her: *New word. Nothing's wicked or mega or kriss anymore; it's all sick – Leo told me.*
Me: *Cool.*
Her: *No!*
Me: *What?*
Her: *No one says cool anymore – so lame.*
Me: (Feeling like a really out-of-touch mother.) *Well, I like*

the bedroom, thank you, and the furniture. (She had gone all out and my savings had suffered.)

Her: *Well, how about it, then?*

Me: *What? Writing? I am!*

Her: *Duh, yeah! But—*

Me: *Wait! Why are you still here?*

Her: *Who cares? Don't wanna go back to that small town anyway! Write the story!*

Me: *What?*

Her: *Yeah, write about what happened to me; peeps have sooooo got to know.*

Me: *Are you serious?*

Her: *As serious as your barf-worthy dress sense! Write the story, my story – no, our story – and tell people.*

Me: (light-bulb flash)

Her: (laughing) *And make sure you write to me and tell me how it all goes!*

This, I believe, is when Teen Nay and I bonded and started to merge. And this was the beginning of everything changing.

Months passed and the writing was keeping me focused. I was putting everything that had happened to me, and to Teen Nay, in order. I still wasn't sure how to deal with my friends, so I used the writing as a reason for my sudden unavailability, until I could figure something out. Through the writing class I found work volunteering on some short-film sets as a prop and set designer and I began to look forward to going to bed and trying to get a good night's sleep, fresh for the next day.

Structure was forming in my life and that structure was slowly revealing a purpose. I was starting to climb out of the black hole that had threatened to consume me for most of my life, and I began to see that perhaps Teen Nay was right. Maybe it wasn't too late for me and I could find my way; find my path, my purpose. But if so, how?

I found that in writing her story, I was gradually starting to see that maybe some positivity could come out of what I had seen as somewhat of a traumatic experience.

And then, in a heartbeat, everything changed again.

Eve came to live in Manchester.

Apart from this one time, when Simone had attempted to build a bridge between us on her graduation day, I hadn't seen Eve properly for almost four years.

And now, because her alcoholism had grown increasingly worse and she was about to lose her job, Simone had invited her to live with her and had offered to help her get into a re-habilitation facility. I was in shock.

Eve moving to Manchester six months after my amnesia made me anxious and conflicted. Part of me wanted to fall into her arms and tell her everything I had been through with the memory loss, but the other part said, *No, don't trust her, this isn't real.*

Simone had told her about the memory loss but I had never asked what Eve had thought about it. I was having a hard enough time with everything that had just happened, fearful it might happen again at any moment. Despite Teen Nay encouraging me to give up smoking, I turned to weed, the only thing I thought would help me cope. But one night, I realized it just wasn't having the same mind-numbing effect it used to.

It was strange seeing Eve for the first time; she had lost a lot of weight and looked pale. I'd gone round to Simone's from the film set where I'd been working to pick up Leo. Eve offered me dinner and we made small talk as I ate. She asked questions about Leo and tried to get to know about my life, but it felt strained, forced almost. I wanted to leave as soon as possible.

When Leo and I got home, I kept thinking about Eve and how disjointed everything seemed. After all but disappearing from my life for fifteen years, had she really returned, attempting to play a role that was no longer necessary? It didn't feel right. I was scared and felt helpless, so called Nat, Marcy and Katie for comfort; they agreed that it wasn't paranoid thinking and that I did have valid reasons not to trust her. Eve was an alcoholic. She had been a functional alcoholic for a long time during my late childhood and adult life and I had learned through years of experience of living with her that what she said, and ultimately what she did, could never really be trusted. It had made things hard because I still loved her unconditionally. But that love meant that I also carried this sense of responsibility, a belief that I had either created or somehow contributed to Eve's alcoholism.

As I had got older, I came to realize that in order for her to continue the cycle of self-abuse, she had to blame everyone, other than herself, for what she did. Sometimes that would include my sister or me. Even though I did everything to make her feel as comfortable as possible, even buying her favourite alcohol and weed when she visited, the blame was always there. Sometimes I would try to have a conversation with her about how worried I was about her drinking but she would always cry and accuse me of judging her. If I asked her advice about something, she would somehow feel that I was blaming her for running off with the postman when I was eighteen and disappearing to London, and she would cry again. I just always felt worse about myself afterwards so stopped trying.

Still, even though I knew the blame was coming, it always hit me like an unexpected slap in the face. After years of this, aged twenty-nine, I couldn't take the stress this unpredictability brought, so I wrote her a long letter explaining how her alcoholism affected me and then I cut her out of my life. This was four years ago and now . . . now she was back and I had no clue how to deal with her.

One night, after a day of prop and set designing on a Blackpool film set, I had told Leo a story and put him to bed. Then, in the quiet house, I tried to think back to the time – around 1993/4, when I was seventeen or eighteen years of age – when I realized my mum was an alcoholic. It was all fuzzy, and as there were no diaries to refer back to, I decided it might help me to write down what I could remember.

29 December 2008

Dear Teen Nay,

Remembering has been difficult because at first I couldn't find one reason as to why, or even when or how it started. But now I realize it has just been a collection of experiences that when grouped together one day made me realize that Eve did have a drink problem. Maybe it is the same for her – that there isn't just one reason why she drinks; maybe it's lots of reasons rolled into one. Maybe.

I remember fragments. Like when I was about seventeen, and me and Sim refused to babysit for the neighbour's kid so that her and Eve could go out together. We had this heated argument, and Simone grabbed a bottle of wine out of the fridge and smashed it on the concrete path in the garden.

And then I realized that all of those times when she would go missing, and we would knock on the neighbours' doors looking for her, finally made sense. She liked to have a good time, she liked to go out, she liked to have a drink. I didn't even mind her drunkenly slapping me across the face and telling me she loved me when she, Aunty Gina and Aunty Becca would return from the club. It was fun watching them dance in the kitchen and make fried egg sandwiches while they laughed with each other about what happened in the shebeens. It all seemed to go very wrong when Joseph left. Her drinking got worse overnight and then she started doing things that were beyond embarrassing. I suppose the smashing of the bottle was Simone's brave protest. At that point, though, I was so detached from my reality. I was leaving to live with Aunty Gina in London and I held so much anger towards Eve for kicking me out because things had gone really wrong in Liverpool with Art and I wasn't speaking to him.

I just wanted to get as far away as possible from everything, including my own mind.

I reckon the pain I was supressing evolved into

*resentment, and every time I went back to
Wolverhampton to visit her and my sister and saw that
her drinking had worsened, I became more detached.
And then when Joseph disappeared, well, she just toppled
over the edge of her grief and fell head first into a barrel
of lager-filled despair, and began to drink every day.*

The more I wrote about my experiences with my mum, the
more I began to unearth all of the negative emotions I had
buried over the years. And as I wrote, I could see exactly when
it was that I had let go of the idea of her ever being a mum to
me.

*I was eighteen and living with Lou, trying to get the
money together to go to Canada, when my ex-boyfriend
– the original emotional vampire – chased me down a set
of stone steps. I fell, he dragged me up off the floor, pinned
me up against a phone box and bit and sucked on my
neck until he left a large red and swollen mark. I was so
distressed and scared that when Eve came up to see Lou
the next day, Lou told her what had happened. Part of
me wanted Eve to go over and slap him up the side of his
drug-addled head. But I think because of her fear of a
situation that probably seemed out of her control, she
drank instead and I got high.*

*That was the day I realized I was no longer her
responsibility and that she was never going to be the
mother that I wanted or needed. Not long after this, I got
so stressed as a result of the stalking, violent, crack-head
Dracula that I lost my two part-time jobs, started taking*

*a lot of ecstasy, acid and speed and eventually had a
nervous breakdown. I went back to live with Art and put
as much physical and emotional distance as I could
between Eve and me. Which was easy considering she
had left to live in London, and had slipped deeper into
her alcoholism.*

*Three years later, when Leo was born, I did try to build
bridges and she would come to Manchester to see us once
a year. But because of her drinking, I began to dread her
visits. They just caused more harm than good.*

*The last chance saloon was when she tried to put
Bacardi Breezer in Leo's Power Ranger cup, claiming it
was like juice. My son was eight! That, together with her
drunken revelation that Art wasn't my real father, pushed
me over the edge. I started to do lots of cocaine and had
my second nervous breakdown. I was twenty-nine.*

*I decided the only thing I could do was to cut her out
of my life for good. And I told everyone who didn't know
me that I was grieving the death of my mother.*

It was the only way I thought I could cope.

*And now she is back and I don't know how to deal. I
really don't know how to deal. I don't know what to do
and I don't want to let you down but I don't know what
to do.*

I need help.
    Adult Naomi x

Writing to her like she had written to me helped me remain
aware that Teen Nay was watching from the sidelines and
it was up to me to protect her. I had to be her Serket now.

She had blamed herself for starting all of this and wanted to make things better, and I was beginning to suspect that she was sticking around to see if I was going to follow through on what she had started. In all of this, me writing our stories was my way of helping her realize that she had been full of potential, although she had buried it seventeen years ago.

And then it all changed. Again.

I had tried, I really had. I even let Simone bring Eve up to my house for dinner a few times. Every time they would come she would bring me flowers, or a nice vase to put them in. So I knew she was trying as well. But I found it awkward and intense. So much had been left unsaid and I wanted to confront her, but felt I couldn't because she was in such a delicate place. I needed something to happen. One night I got what I had asked for.

Missing her company and desperate to spend some time alone with her, I called Simone to see if she wanted to go to watch a film at the cinema. Just the two of us. Leo was already staying at her house and she asked Eve to keep an eye on him for a couple of hours. I was reticent at first; Eve was acting excitable and I suspected she may have already been drinking that day. But I didn't want to accuse her and for her to feel victimized.

Leo was outside playing with his friends when I arrived, so I quietly told him that if anything happened he should go to Simone's friend Marianne's house and she would call me straight away.

I suppose I wanted to let Eve see that in spite of everything that had happened, I could still make attempts to trust her.

My attempts were in vain. When we arrived back from the cinema, I checked on Leo, who was still playing at his friend's house.

'Just letting you know I'm back, son.' I popped my head round the bedroom door, seeing he was on the PlayStation with his friend Tom. Leo nodded.

'Everything okay?' I asked him.

'Yeah, but Nanna was acting funny.'

My heart started to pulse. 'Funny how?' I already knew he meant she was drunk.

He turned from the screen, gave me a sweet smile and shrugged. 'You know, weird funny.'

'Oh, okay.' I took a deep breath. 'Well, I'm at Sim's now so I'll come and get you when we're ready to go,' I told him.

'Okay.' He turned back to the screen and continued to play.

By the time I had walked the breadth of the gated complex, the fear I felt had pulled memories of betrayal from the dark recesses of my mind and pushed me over the edge into rage. I stormed into Simone's living room. 'Have you been drinking?' I shouted at Eve.

'Nay, calm down,' Simone interjected.

'Calm down? Calm fucking down? Are you kidding me, Simone? The one chance . . .' I turned to Eve. 'The one chance I give you and this is what you do? How dare you get drunk while looking after my child!'

'Nay.' Simone stepped closer to me.

Eve stood up. 'So?' she shouted back, slurring a bit. 'You don't understand. I didn't even want to babysit, I wanted to come with you two.'

'What? Why didn't you say something?' Simone asked her.

'You didn't ask,' she said, tears welling in her eyes. 'I don't even want to be here. I fucking hate this place!'

'So why the bloody hell are you here?' I said. 'Pack up your suitcase and go back to London.'

'I can't.' She moved over to the window and started to cry. 'They don't want me there anymore. They said that I'm an alcoholic, that I needed to come here, but I don't even want to be here.'

'Oh, boo hoo for you.' I saw red, taking what she had just said as a sign of ungratefulness for all that Simone had done for her. 'I'm so sorry that you have to come and spend some actual real time with your family.'

I then went into a tirade, yelling that I'd been telling her for years that she had a drink problem, and that it was a sad state of affairs that it took her boss's family telling her to make her act, rather than her listening to her own children. Simone tried to calm things down, but I went ballistic at her. I had finally reached my limit and everything I had ever wanted to say flew out of my mouth, backed by an awful rage.

'You're irresponsible,' I screamed at her, 'and selfish, and for years it's always been about you, while me and Simone have been left to defend ourselves!' I slapped my chest hard, accentuating every word.

'Well, you don't understand! The life I've had, the things I've been through, my mum . . .' she cried.

'Oh my God, get over yourself, woman. We've all had fucked-up things happen to us, and I can match you on dysfunctional mothers,' I yelled, 'but there comes a time when you have to take responsibility for your actions; you can't keep bloody blaming everyone for the choices that YOU make.'

We went round in circles, for hours, me accusing her of playing the victim and how tired it was getting, her defending herself in true Amy Winehouse style, stating that she didn't want to stop drinking or go to rehab (no, no, no) and Simone trying to calm the situation down.

Eventually Simone rubbed her forehead in exasperation. 'Nay, Mum, there's no point us going over the same stuff again and again. You're both hurting, we are all hurting, but we need to find a way to move forward; we need to find a solution. Mum.' She turned to Eve, who at this point was crying and smoking a cigarette by the window. 'I understand you don't want to be here, and yeah, it's not ideal living with me, but I am trying to help you, and what's the alternative? You go back to London and then what? They are not going to give you your job back. They love and care about you and want you to get better; at least think about getting better first and maybe you can go back to London then.'

Simone took a deep breath and turned to me. 'Nay, I know you're angry, and you have every right to be, and not just about tonight. I've seen how stuff Eve's said and done has affected you, you're valid in how you feel, but it's late and we aren't getting anywhere. Why don't you get Leo and go home.'

She was right. Arguing with someone who was drunk didn't make any sense and I couldn't see a resolution; I just wanted Eve to leave. But I realized at that point that I was exhausted and remembered it was a school night. It was way past Leo's bedtime.

I drove home, and after putting an already sleeping Leo to bed, I sat downstairs until the early hours of the morning, finally seeing the connection between my fractured relationship with my mother and my fractured sense of self. I tried to smoke but it just made me feel really sick. In the end I realized that what I was feeling was a deep sadness. I hadn't felt good about any of the things I had said. In fact, I just felt sorry for all of us, and the whole painful situation. We had all been trapped in a powerful triangle for years and the roles that we had played had crept back up on us: Eve the victim, Simone the rescuer and me the villain. Over the years we had exchanged roles, but I knew one thing for sure: we had all been stuck in a situation that was no longer working for any of us and it had finally come to an explosive end.

As I was getting Leo ready for school the next morning, I received a text from Simone telling me that Eve had run away the night before and had gone on a drinking binge. I was angry. And underneath this anger was fear, and this fear battled with the underlying guilt I felt for saying what I had the previous night to my mum. After years of feeling bad about speaking my mind to her, and feeling that I was doing something wrong and that was why she drank, I so desperately wanted to feel different – different about her, different about myself. It was too painful. I wanted things to change for the better. Perhaps that explains what happened next.

28 February 2009

Dear Teen Nay,

I've just had a blazing row with Simone. I don't even know half the things I said to her; I was just crying and shouting down the phone at her.

After the argument the other night, Eve ran away on a drinking binge.

Late yesterday she was found fallen down drunk on the ground by a couple. They went through the small phone book she had on her and phoned Simone. She tried to prepare me but I was still mortified when I saw her face. I swear she looked like she had gone ten rounds with Mike Tyson. I half expected to find her ear bitten off, she was so unrecognizable. Her top lip was bloodied and cut and had swelled to twice its size, a deep purple and red colour ringed her left eye, and one side of her face was grazed red. It looked like the pavement had tried to take the top layer of her skin off. The couple had said she was very drunk and incoherent and they thought she had been beaten and left for dead.

You know what? There was a part of me that wanted to burst into tears and run to her side, hugging her and apologizing for what I had said the night before. But instead I stood and stared at her, searching for a hint of insincerity behind her swollen eyes while she cried and apologized. The ever-compassionate Simone tried to encourage me to hug her but I just looked at my mum incredulously and drank my tea. A disgust that she would do this to herself and a despair that my sister had brought her and her drama back into our lives coursed through me, and you know what? I felt no compassion for her. Empathy has evaded me. All I could think was, I want her to go home. I want her to leave and go back to her little bedsit in London and drown in her drink and misery and leave me, and my son, out of it. *Simone said under no circumstances was she sending her back and*

*she had every intention of helping Eve get sober and
encouraging her to stay in Manchester.*

*This morning, I woke up thinking I just couldn't take it
anymore and I have just got off the phone to Sim and told
her I would never forgive her for bringing Eve here.*

*I think somewhere deep down inside of me I know I
have created this situation, created the argument, because
I need a way out of feeling responsible for Eve and her
alcoholism.*

I just needed a way out.
> *Love,*
> *Adult Naomi x*

To try and make sense of all of this, I turned to the dissertation I had written when I was in the homeless hostel. It was
about adult children of alcoholics and their coping strategies
or, in my case, their lack thereof.

According to a source quoted in my dissertation, 'Adult
children of alcoholics often have dysfunctional childhoods
which provide them with few or no "normal life" experiences,
so they guess at what correct behaviour is to stop others from
discovering that they genuinely don't know how they should
act, react, talk or simply be. Their feelings about themselves
are the opposite of the serene image they present – they generally feel insecure, inadequate, dull, unsuccessful, vulnerable,
unlovable and anxious.'*

Apparently, because of my 'maladaptive coping strategies',

---

* Woititz, J. G. (1983) *Adult Children of Alcoholics* (Hollywood, FL: Health
Communications, Inc.).

I was destroying any adult ability I possessed to develop a healthy mature identity. The narrative went on to say that adult children of alcoholics were often self-protective people-pleasers, who sought approval from others while risking the loss of their own identities in the process. This also made sense to me. I was this adult child and I had lost my identity. I lacked the coping resources for dealing with life events, which, according to what I read, was me modelling the alcoholic parent's strategies, which included avoidance and escape-related tactics. I couldn't help but see the irony.

The following weeks I closed off, became more withdrawn. I also stopped speaking to Simone. After our argument, I didn't want any contact with her or Eve. I was too angry, hurt and upset by everything that had happened.

I retreated into my cocoon and placed my mind in that warm, safe, imaginary world I had known as a child. I became Edna the Storyteller again (minus the frillies on my head) and I wrote stories where I created characters who did and said what I wanted them to and where I could invent all the happy endings I wished.

I was so conflicted and confused that at times I felt like I wanted to lose myself. My mind wanted to repeat the same pattern of splitting again, to take on the familiar role of the abused and abandoned child, and then split again into the adult who wanted a better life. Except this time something was different – I had Teen Nay and I could feel her willing me to stay where I was.

To my surprise, Dean, Katie, Marcy and Nat were support-ive of me not seeing Simone or Eve, encouraging me to talk to them whenever I needed to.

I felt trapped in a pattern from childhood, which translated into me believing with such conviction that I didn't matter. That no matter how I felt or no matter how much a person claimed to love me, in the end something would always happen (the violence or the abuse) that reinforced the premise of the story of my life.

I don't matter.

So I swapped joints for Krispy Kremes and wrote about my past and my life with Eve and Simone. The more I wrote, the more I indulged a part of my psyche that emerged through the written words on the page – that of ten-year-old Naomi. Ten years of age was the second time in my life I was sexually abused and when I had my very first cigarette.

I felt as if my life was like a long Tennessee Williams play. A memory play, in which the character experiences an occurrence in the present that dredges up an overwhelming trauma from the past and causes time to form a kind of loop so this character cannot escape the present until they escape the past.

Then the film production company emailed me and asked me if I could work on the last of the four films I had signed up to help with.

Immersion was an abstract short film about the loss of languages across the world, exploring how each generation was speaking less and less in their mother tongue and losing the connection to their history and their ancestry. The main character was a French girl, Angelique, and the director, Roberta, was an artist by profession who was very focused on the cinematography. I loved her passion and her infectious need to realize her own vision. We shot the film in Liverpool, the city where I was born. And as I watched it being filmed, I realized *Immersion* was essentially about death.

In one scene Angelique had to stand with her eyes closed so that Roberta could create the illusion that the crowd walking past her was walking in fast motion while Angelique was completely still in real time. It was a cold March day, so I stood off-camera, on hand with coats and blankets to provide some warmth when filming stopped. During one break, as I approached the actress, I noticed something on her tights. It was a beautiful green and speckled blue butterfly, a strange sight for a cold winter's day. The butterfly allowed me to take it from her leg and place it on her hand. Miraculously, it didn't fly away. We called Roberta over and she immediately captured it on film, the butterfly, sitting peacefully in the palm of the actress's hand. It completed the scene and we could not see it as anything other than fate, because when she finished the shot, she tried to pick the butterfly from Angelique's hand and it flew away.

A comforting peace descended on the crew on the drive back to Roberta's apartment, where she provided lunch. I couldn't stop thinking about the butterfly and I didn't know why until later, when we were shooting a scene in Roberta's small kitchen. We didn't need a full crew, so there were only four of us there, waiting for Angelique to get ready. Billy, the boom operator, was setting up the microphone. Chris, the cameraman, was fixing the tripod and I was placing the necessary culinary items on the table. Roberta was looking through the camera, talking through her angles and shots. All of a sudden she shouted: 'Oh my god, my mum!' We all looked to where she was pointing the camera. It was a beautiful black-and-white picture of a white-haired, slim-faced, pretty woman, an almost angelic light captured in her eyes.

Roberta burst into tears and slumped to the floor. I knew instantly that her mother had died and although the picture of her had most probably been there all this time, looking through the lens of a camera meant that she had somehow seen it for the first time. Everyone froze. I stepped to her, crouched to the floor, and hugged her, telling her everything would be okay.

I felt her grief. I thought of all the people I had loved who had either disappeared from my life or died, and I knew that loss could hit you in the most unlikeliest of places at the most unlikeliest of times. It turned out Roberta had lost her mother only weeks before and as professional and composed as she was, the grief eventually spilled out.

And as I hugged her, I understood that we were all immersed in a time of loss and it became clear what the butterfly was telling us. Life is short, relationships end, you lose people; you go through a lot of pain and hard times. Everything changes; it's a given. You grow, only to experience everything fading: your memories, even your language, and the connection you have to the people you thought would be in your life forever. But you have to be like the butterfly on Angelique's palm, fighting for your place, fighting for your purpose, standing strong against a harsh, cold wind. And in order to truly live your life, you have to experience the loss, the death itself, to realize your true self, who you really are.

I felt as she watched from the house of my mind that this experience had helped Teen Nay understand the future world that she thought was a tragedy. She began to see that in order to embrace the new, the world had to experience the death of the old. Lose a language today, and create a new one tomorrow. Create a global language. Make it digital. For some it would be painful; for others it would be progress.

Was *Immersion* telling me I needed to do this to make way for the new? Was Eve's appearance just another indicator that it was time to let go of the other parts of me that had got stuck in the past? If so, then maybe her turning up wasn't necessarily a bad thing. Maybe it was time. If I could handle seventeen years of memory loss, then maybe I could handle anything.

Maybe.

Roberta was a stranger to me, but for that split second, I experienced her vulnerability and loss, and wanted to comfort her. As I held her to me, it finally helped me to feel compassion for Eve and all the grief and loss she was experiencing. I knew then that if I truly wanted change, if I wanted to let go, I had to let myself experience my pain rather than trying to escape from it, even though it was going to hurt. Firstly, I had to stop it being all about Eve and stop waiting for the mother I never had. I had to accept that I was my own mother and I could give birth to a new me and raise her to be the emotionally strong, healthy woman I wanted to be. Secondly, while I knew giving birth was painful, this time around, I had to do it without any drugs.

13

Au Revoir, Paris

*It's not how everyone
looks at you,
but how you look at yourself.
How are you looking at yourself?
With eyes in blindness or eyes of kindness?*

I. J.

'Transient Global Amnesia?'
  'Yes.'
  'Transient Global Amnesia?'
  'That's the one.'
  'For how long?'
  'Well, eight weeks.'

My memories had fully returned, and given the level of change the amnesia had brought, I felt like I needed a few months for it to all sink in. But once it had, I knew I needed to go to my doctor and see if he could help me. He listened intently and then turned to the computer. My last visit had been noted: 'Patient presented with memory loss, due to pressure from exams; reassured and sent home.'

He didn't say a word, just rose from his chair, opened his door, and left the room. He returned a few moments later with a strained smile on his face.

I didn't know where he had disappeared to; it could have been to the toilet. But I told myself it had something to do with that Doctor Davies' complete disregard for me. You don't just tell a patient who is sitting opposite you telling you they are fifteen again to go home and have a cup of tea. Not with my history!

Doctor Rahman was apologetic and assured me that he would do everything in his power to make sure this didn't happen again. He wasn't too alarmed because my memories had by now mostly returned. I told him that I was determined not to go through this again and needed to understand exactly what had happened to my brain. I asked him to refer me to a psychiatrist and he recommended we get in touch with the social worker who had helped me when I'd been homeless two years earlier. As a consequence, I left the surgery feeling more in control of a situation that had controlled me for far too long. As soon as I got home, I binned the prescription he had given me. I wanted to show Teen Nay that I could learn how to be my own antidepressant.

Things started to change, slowly, subtly, quietly. Still, there was one last thing I had to do.

Even though for Teen Nay the story had started the moment she woke up in the future – my future – what had happened before my memory loss was still haunting me. My story had started in Paris, from the moment I'd met Henri, the 'French Dude' with whom I had had a passionate, whirlwind romance. It was the break-up with him that had been the final push for me to stop caring about my life. In my despair, I'd yet again felt there was no point trying to make good things happen because no matter what, I always failed. Of course, his ex-girlfriend turning up at his flat to 'talk' to me at one o'clock in the morning and me realizing I had walked into a messy break-up had a lot to do with it. But the stomach virus and tonsillitis I contracted after this had happened obscured my judgement and I, as Teen Nay put it, blamed myself for '*other people's mental tosser issues*'.

So even after all I'd been through, I still thought about him. We were Facebook friends but our correspondence was polite, with the odd comment on each other's status. We had gone from being in a short, intense relationship to being virtual strangers and as much as I pretended I was okay with it, I wasn't . . . at first.

Cue this conversation with Teen Nay while sitting at the computer one day:

Her: (Sticking fingers down throat) *Bluurrgh!!*
Me: *But—*
Her: *No, no, no, no! This is sooooo wack. He is, like, ignoring you!*
Me: *But he is still watering my crops and feeding my chickens for me on my virtual farm.*
Her: *Seriously?! Park up the combine harvester, get out and get over it!*
Me: *But—*
Her: *Erm, exsqueeze me! He'd rather milk your virtual cows than talk to you? Sad, sad, saddo, sad! Saaaaaddddddd!!*

I closed the laptop.

She was right. If I wanted to let go of the old Naomi, I needed to let go of the ways I was used to relating to men – especially the unhealthy pattern I'd developed of looking for my self-worth in men who rescued me or fed my virtual pigs.

So the universe answered Teen Nay's prayers and when I reopened the laptop, I saw an email from my old friend Georgie! She was coming back!

Georgina and I had met at university. As soon as she walked into the room, I noticed her. There was something about her. She was beautiful, yes, but there was something else, something intangible that others saw too. Some people hated her for it; others were intimidated by it or jealous. I loved it. Georgina had what I simply liked to call 'It'.

She was genuinely interested in others and made you feel like her focus was on you and only you, and that she saw into your soul and believed that you were a good person who deserved the best. I found when I watched her talk to people that this somehow morphed into a spirited, sexy, outspoken confidence and an air of erudition that would make the smartest man crumble into an insensible heap. She seemed to travel in her very own constellation and took her rightful place at the centre of it. The brightest star in the sky. Georgie could also kick butt on the Nintendo, bake lovely cakes, and make a mean Margarita.

Fed up with the mundane nine-to-five routine after university, Georgie had decided to rent out her flat for several months and travel the world on a cruise ship. During my amnesia, she had been somewhere in the middle of the Pacific, partying in spectacular style with gorgeous-tasting cocktails and even more gorgeous-looking men. She'd been completely unaware of what I was going through, but as soon as she arrived home I was the first person she contacted. Leo was at home with Art and JJ so I drove over to her apartment, desperate to tell her everything.

As soon as I saw Georgina standing there, as fabulous as always in her Jimmy Choo shoes, health radiating from every pore of her sun-kissed ochre-brown skin, I burst into tears of joy and hugged her until my arms ached. She was still gorgeous Georgie, with her adorable smile, and her oriental-shaped eyes still had that cheeky twinkle.

It was great to have her back. I realized how much I had missed her and, to my delight, Teen Nay thought she was '*top bananas*'. Sitting at the table with a couple of bottles of Merlot, she entertained me with tales from her adventures at sea, giggling about the 'adoring men' who wanted to marry her and whisk her off into a life of champagne and yachts. She was fabulous and the one female friend (apart from Katie) that Teen Nay approved of. We had a truly synergetic relationship – protective of each other and able to confide in each other whenever we needed.

And so it was within no time at all that she decided we needed a weekend away and that in order for me to get closure on the past and the amnesia, we should go to Paris, the place where the story had started for me.

It was also a great excuse to go and see Beyoncé, one of her all-time favourite artists. She was not really my cup of tea – if I did crave music with soul, I turned to the greats, like Aretha, Al and Marvin – but I soon got into her songs. I found Georgina's school of *B'Day* enlightening – although I did wonder about naming an album after an arse-washing sink – and I enjoyed singing along and dancing to her songs and revelling in America's answer to girl-power-type music, with an R&B flavour.

I was even more taken with Beyoncé and her vocal skills when I heard her rendition of 'Ave Maria'. I definitely wanted to see her live, so made arrangements with Art to have Leo for the weekend and Georgie and I booked two concert tickets, two plane tickets, and hotel rooms for a weekend in Paris.

Georgie and I missed our flight because we spent too long in the airport lounge eating noodles and drinking wine. We found this hilarious and rebooked ourselves on the next flight. But by the time I got on the next plane I wondered if it was a bad sign. From the bedroom window of the house of my mind, a watchful Teen Nay rolled her eyes.

As soon as we reached Paris, everything came flooding back and I wasn't sure if I was doing the right thing. On the Metro I saw me holding hands with Henri on a speeding train, listening to French love songs on his iPod. When we arrived at the hotel, I saw his small apartment with its wooden floors and rickety cast-iron lift, as if I were there again. I lay in bed wondering whether he was lying in his bed thinking about me. Teen Nay just rolled her eyes.

The day of the concert was strange, like *Twilight Zone* strange. I had only one desire, to walk down the Champs-Élysées. Even though I'd been to the city a few times I had never stepped foot on the famous road, full of incredibly expensive boutiques. Georgie and I changed from one metro station to another and finally arrived in an arrondissement that we thought would take us there. A pretty French woman laughed at us when we asked her whether we were anywhere near. In broken English, she explained we had somehow managed to get ourselves over to the other side of the city. This reminded me of the last time I had been lost in Paris and how I'd needed a man (a policeman at that) to rescue me.

'What is it with me, my internal GPS and Paris?' I said to Georgie. 'I've been all over the world and it's the only place I seem to get lost in.'

'Babe, it really doesn't matter, we're here!' Georgie stuck her button nose in the air, ignoring the peremptoriness Paris seemed to possess. 'Let's go and eat canapés and drink champagne.'

Admittedly, by then I was growing tired of looking over my shoulder all the time, worrying that I was going to bump into Henri on every street corner, so a glass of champagne sounded like heaven. This drink and several more afterwards made us late for the concert and we ended up in the middle of a large crowd made up of predominantly French teenagers waiting for Beyoncé to come on stage. Needless to say, having just starred in my own version of *My So-Called Life* – having been fifteen TWICE! – I had little patience for sweating, hormonal, screaming adolescents.

I was crushed into a very small space, grabbing hold of my bag furiously in case any one of the little thugs tried to rob my euros. It was taking a lot for me not to fall into a high-heeled sweaty heap on the floor. I eventually had no choice but to turn to Teen Nay, who was standing with arms folded and, yes, rolling her eyes at me from the window of the house of my mind.

Her: *Are you, like, for real? You are not a victim; you need to*
  get a grip, seriously!
Me: *I know. I'm just not comfortable; I want to go home.*
Her: *Since when did not being comfortable ever stop us? Stop*
  you? Why are you so bloody scared of everything? This is,
  like, beyond stale; this is . . . just who are you, woman?
  Get a life! Jeez!

She was right; it had been nearly a year since the amnesia
and she was watching me, and I was watching her watching
me and still seeing everything from her eyes. It wasn't good.
I could feel myself slowly slipping into my debilitating fears
again. I was beginning to use the fact that I still wasn't speaking to Simone and Eve as a big red stamp on the contract of
my failed life.

Gosh, I was at a concert – a concert! – and I was freaking out
because I was getting squashed. In writing to Teen Nay I had
found parts of me that I had buried: the survivor, the fighter
and the diva. She had made one thing clear to me: that no
matter what I experienced in life, I could, and always would,
survive and adapt. Now I took a deep breath and inhaled her
thoughts, which provided me with a little push of courage. I
threw off my heels and put on my spare flats. I grabbed a pop
sock out of my bag, tied a knot in it and scraped back my hair.
I took the scarf from around my neck, wiped my brow and
tied the handles of my bag, securing it. I pushed to the left
of me, to the right of me, in front of me and behind, letting
the unsuspecting teens know that I was rightfully claiming
my space and was willing to go down fighting – no, defending it. And then everything was forgotten as soon as Beyoncé

glided across the stage all glittered and glamorous, belting out powerful songs about independent women and putting rings on it.

She was incredible, beautiful, and mesmerizing. I hung off her every word and marvelled at every dance move. I swam in a sea of soulful cries, heartfelt laments and uplifting melodies, and listened to lyrics that spoke to my heart and helped take my own thoughts to a better, more peaceful place, no more so than when she walked onto the stage, dressed all in white, singing 'Ave Maria' with an azure blue sea in the background. The colours reminded me of Egypt and a flowing sense of freedom came to me.

'Here's your song, Nay,' Georgie shouted to me across the crowd.

As Beyoncé sang, her dancers surrounded her and covered her from head to toe in a silk and lace white wedding dress with a veil. I couldn't help but think of all of the men I had tried to have relationships with while wounded and the tears flowed. I didn't care who was watching me (although I'm sure not many were, considering an international pop star was on the stage). I sobbed to the operatic-esque song where she sang about a little girl being lost, hurt and lonely, and some-times not fitting in, but knowing there was someone always watching over her. It made me think of my teenage self, splitting seventeen years ago but coming back to my future with a ferocious insistence that I mattered, that I deserved a good life.

The image of this singer standing there, the virginal bride waiting for the one to come and take her hand, allowed me to weep for that same image I had always held of me, this little girl lost in the darkness waiting for some light to come and hold my hand. I cried deep healing tears the whole time she sang that song. I was letting go of the belief that I needed rescuing and releasing the need to base my identity on victimhood.

As she floated across the stage and the dress moved with her soft steps, the blue spotlights illuminated it and bathed her in a cerulean glow. I realized it was I who had done the abandoning. I had disapproved of my true desires – and myself – giving in to what others wanted and expected of me and not what I wanted and needed. Naomi Jacobs had lost Naomi Jacobs and Teen Nay had come back to find her. To find me. She had whisked me away to my own blue skies and azure seas and taken me on a journey so deep inside myself that I could no longer deny my true self. Myself as soul. Myself as body. Myself as a precious and delicate broken mind that needed healing.

The song reached a crescendo and the soprano notes vibrated across the silent crowd. I knew then that every man I had ever met in my adult life was the one for me, but only for the time he was supposed to be, and it was meant to end when it did. The pain came from me trying to hold on to something that was no longer meant for me. I wasn't coming back to Paris to let go of Henri. I was coming back to Paris to let go of a twenty-seven-year-old belief that was no longer working for me: the belief that I was a victim and the only time I was worth something to anyone was when I was being rescued.

As the dancers took Beyoncé's hands and led her up the steps towards the great wall of baby blue sky and white clouds,

I believed with a sudden clarity that when I did eventually meet another man, I wouldn't feel like a victim and need rescuing. I would be brave and loving and would take care of myself. Our relationship wouldn't start off with me playing damsel in distress and him pulling out his sword (ahem) and charging to the rescue. No, we would meet as equals, regardless of what we had been through and the scars we carried; we would see them as a testament of our strength and not as a weakness. We would celebrate that in each other, not fear it, label it, and hide from it. I knew I needed this in my friendships also.

Just because someone had come along and unbalanced it all once didn't mean that I, Naomi Jacobs, couldn't find the balance again. Find the feminine, the woman in me, the child, the teenager and the mother all working together to heal me, complementing and providing me with the strength and love that I needed to nourish my self-worth and self-confidence.

To nourish me.

The last notes of 'Ave Maria' died away and the stage grew dark. Whilst standing there, wiping my tears, I knew that I also needed to embrace the dark side of myself. It was the part where fear came from but also the part of myself that put up a fight, defending my corner. I needed to accept the shadows that had hidden the destructive side, to overcome the voice that told me I couldn't cope without some mind-altering substance. If I could accept the shadow, then maybe I could let it go. Stop its power over me.

While the crowd cheered and screamed for more I thought back to a few hours earlier in the hotel room where I had whinged about the excess weight I'd put on since quitting smoking and falling into a vat of Green & Black's chocolate. Georgie did everything to convince me that with my small breasts, slim waist and curvy hips and thighs, I still looked great. I'd stood in front of the mirror, glaring at my body, disgusted that I had let myself go.

She had jumped off the bed and grabbed my arms. 'Right, put your hands here.' I put my hands at the side of my body by my breasts. 'Now,' she continued. 'With your hands still attached to your body, slide them down as far as they can go.' I'd giggled nervously as I traced my body shape and pulled my hands away when I reached my waist.

'No, no, I can't; this is daft.' I'd felt stupid and turned away from the mirror, closing my eyes in shame. Georgie grabbed my shoulders and turned me back to the mirror.

'No, look, you have to embrace your body, your shape. You're not unhealthy or obese. You're gorgeous, babe. You are sexy. But only you can tell yourself this.' She put my hands on my waist. 'Carry on,' she commanded. I did and took a deep breath, nodding in agreement. After all, some women did this every day; what was the big deal in moving your hands across your body in appreciation of your figure? I had done it before many times on my own. However, I hadn't realized that doing it fully clothed in front of a mirror, in front of my best friend, would bring up so many feelings of shame and embarrassment. When my hands reached my hips, I burst into tears and hung my head down in shame. 'I can't. I'm sorry. I don't think I'm sexy. It doesn't look sexy to me. I don't feel sexy; I feel fat,' I sobbed.

Georgie rushed over and gave me a big hug. 'It's okay, Nay. But seriously, you've got to find a way to love your body. Do you know how sad it is that so many women and young girls hate their bodies because we all think we are supposed to live up to this unrealistic ideal? No matter what shape you are, you have to know that you are a desirable, sensual and sexy woman.'

Teen Nay looked on with sadness, thinking about all of those magazines she read when she woke up in the future with the size-zero airbrushed models.

Maybe it was the abuse my body had suffered at the hands of others and then at my own hands. Maybe it was the familiar rejection I'd felt from Henri ignoring me. Maybe it was the waist on my jeans tightening every day. Or maybe it was the failed relationships with my friends and the ever-widening gap between me and my sister. Whatever it was, it was contributing to me feeling awful about myself, and even more so about my body.

But something changed while I was standing there at the concert. Teen Nay reminded me of the way she had flirted with all of the men on holiday in Egypt and of the date with Ahmed. She had shown me that I needed to honour the part of my womanhood that was sexual and sensual, that it was safe to enjoy my body and express myself in all my curves, dimples and love handles.

When she'd had control of my body, Teen Nay had realized that it hadn't let me down, that it was my friend, that it had protected me. I knew then at the concert that it was okay to let go of that deep feeling of physical inadequacy. It was okay for me to embrace whatever changes my body was going through. I had to start somewhere, and harbouring feelings of hatred towards my body had to stop.

The lights came back on and Beyoncé began another song. As I watched this beautiful athlete twirl and turn gracefully across the stage I knew that I needed to embrace the curves and contours of my life if I was to move as easily in my life as she did in her body, regardless of the size. I took my hands and, starting from the side of my breasts, I traced the curve of my shape and shook my hips in the middle of a crowd of people in a concert in Paris. Teen Nay was right. My body hadn't betrayed me; it had stood by me. It had taken all of the bruises and the batterings and the abuses and was still working for me. My body was my faithful friend and there was no need for me to fear its strength any longer.

I stood proud when the song ended and I wiped away the last of the tears. I felt like I had finally said goodbye to the pain of past relationships that never really stood a chance because they were so unequal in the beginning. I had been hurting for far too long, especially in my relationship with myself.

As I danced the rest of the night away and sung along to even more songs of love and female empowerment, I let go piece by piece, lyric by lyric, note by note, the childhood fantasy of the handsome prince sitting atop a great white horse galloping in to rescue me from a dark and oppressive place. I let go of the need to be married and wear a ring on my finger to feel secure. I let go of the need to have babies to validate my femininity and the desire to mother others to give me a sense of self-worth. I let go of feeling bad about myself if I didn't look like the women in the fashion magazines and on the billboards. I let go of believing I couldn't cope with life or a crisis unless I had a drug to help me along the way. I let go of the old and stated to the world I was ready for the new, and I especially let go of thinking that the only thing I ever deserved to feel like was a victim.

And this time, Teen Nay didn't roll her eyes. She fist-pumped and then mentally high-fived me.

14

The Voice

*At the centre of your being
you have the answer.
You know who you are
And you know what you want.*

LAO-TZU

It was time to pick up the cerebral shovel and start digging.

When I came back from Paris, I knew that if I truly wanted to heal my mind, I would have to do what Teen Nay had said to Ahmed. I had to get out what had broken my mind in the first place. Therapy hadn't fully worked for me in the past. Every time I felt as if I'd had a breakthrough, the sessions would end and I would be left to figure things out for myself. It always felt like I was taking two steps forward and five back. But now I knew it was my only way forward and after having ten therapists over the past ten years, I felt like this was going to be my final attempt.

I had seen my therapist Maria before and was glad that my doctor managed to refer me to her again. It took a couple of weeks after I started for me to open up – I mean, really open up – but when I did, it was like the crack in the dam of my mind couldn't hold and I had to let it break. It all came flooding out. To anyone that would listen – mainly Nat and Marcy and Maria. It took a while for me to trust Maria again so I followed Teen Nay's example and trusted myself. I wanted to discuss my memory loss with her; I wanted to tell her about the diaries, especially what Teen Nay had written and how I was seeing myself so differently now; I wanted to talk about the breakdown of my relationship – again – with my sister and Eve, but not knowing how she would react, I approached therapy carefully at first, revealing things slowly.

All of this cautiousness went out of the window, however, at my long-awaited assessment with yet another psychiatrist whom I was waiting to see while I was having the therapy with Maria. I knew he wasn't an expert in memory loss, but I did think he might be able to help me, or at least explain to me what had happened. Having at first been assigned a trainee assistant who asked me the same questions I had been asked over and over again for the past ten years, I stormed into his office, demanding he see me. He informed me, rather condescendingly, that I had been misdiagnosed with bipolar disorder and that I smoked too much weed. I got scared, then angry, and told him his estimation of my mental state was downright unprofessional.

His 'diagnosis' didn't help. If anything, it only served in having me further question my sanity, the split episodes, and the amnesia. I knew that drugs could exacerbate psychosis, even bring on periods of manic depression. I knew that alcohol impaired a mind's ability to function properly. Any abuse

of a substance would eventually affect the mind. But to completely dismiss my issues and attribute them to a joint was, I
felt, ignorant and arrogant.

I needed answers. He was no help and even though I asked
him whether the sexual, physical and emotional abuse I had
been through, my experience of violence in the home during
my formative years, having to deal with an alcoholic parent,
or my parents abandoning me at crucial developmental ages
had had anything to do with it, he couldn't give me a straight
answer. No, the breakdown of my relationships and the crip-
pling sense of failure I had felt for most of my life was all down
to ganja!

Anyway, all of this came out in an indignant tirade to
Maria one day when I told her in no uncertain terms that I'd
'bloody well had enough of the mental health services and
their inability to properly diagnose me'. After all I'd been
through I felt I had more insight and could do a better job
than they did.

To my surprise, Maria agreed with me, and this helped
stem the flow of anger. We went on to discuss the symptoms
and causes of each possible diagnosis, starting with bipolar
disorder, moving on to dissociative identity disorder and the
'fragmentation of a personality', and ending up at transient
global amnesia. We agreed that every gnarled branch of that
knotted tree stemmed from the roots of abuse and my mind
doing its best to deal with it, to give a name to it, regardless of
whether doctors understood this or not.

Maria's reverence for the power of the mind was passionate and frank.

'Just because it's the mind and you can't see it, feel it or touch it like you can, say, a hand, it doesn't mean it isn't real,' she told me, 'and it doesn't mean that it doesn't get hurt, cut, broken or burnt, or that those wounds are not real and they don't need healing. They do.'

'So what about the split episodes?' I asked her. 'My mind has split on many occasions, the most powerfully when I was six, fifteen, twenty-nine and last year, when I was thirty-two.'

'Well, I think maybe we should go back to the house.'

'I'm not sure,' I said. 'The house of my mind is still there, but something is different.'

'Okay, what if you don't actually go back into it, but sort of revisit the memory of the house and all that you went through in it?' Maria suggested.

I closed my eyes. I looked for the house. It had become almost like a faint outline, an old imprint of itself. Teen Nay was still there, still in her room. But she was waiting, watching, silent and calm, as the walls around her started to fade. She had been growing increasingly quiet since Paris.

'I don't feel like I need to go inside,' I said.

'You don't have to, Naomi, but I want you to look at it and tell me what that house means to you.' Maria's voice was soft, hypnotic almost.

I looked at the house for a while. I felt scared at first, but sitting there with Maria by my side, I was suddenly overcome by a feeling that everything was going to be all right. I remembered it was my house and nobody could get in without my permission.

'Security,' I said. 'Safety. Yes, this is my safe house.'

'A safe house,' Maria repeated.

'I suppose it is. I always felt safe when I put myself in this

house, even though I was scared of what I would find in the
rooms. But,' I said, 'it always in some way seemed to turn out
okay. Once I found the room, the answer, I eventually turned
it around and redecorated.' I laughed and opened one eye.
Maria was smiling,

'So it was a safe house?' she repeated.

'Definitely.'

'Safe from what?' Maria's mellifluous voice seemed to urge
me to look further, deeper.

I stopped focusing on the house for a moment and it all
went dark. 'Safe from the people that could hurt me – no, that
did hurt me. Safe from the pain of what they did, safe from
the world, safe from the enemy.' I opened my eyes again. I
hadn't meant to say 'the enemy', but it had come out of my
mouth nonetheless.

'Enemy?' she echoed.

'Yeah, I suppose so, like a war. It's like I've been fighting a
war for years, in my mind, and those that hurt me have been
the enemy and the house that I built was the safe house – no,
a hospital, or a safe house with a medical room in it – where
I would retreat and try and deal with the wounds. I always
thought my mind was the place of problems, but it's actually
been a sanctuary.'

'It's interesting you use these particular words, war, enemy,
sanctuary,' she remarked. 'Some people who have fought in
wars, physical wars, can suffer some form of post-traumatic
stress disorder.'

'Oh, Jeez! Another disorder; how many can a woman have?'
I joked.

She smiled. 'Well, from what you have been through in

your life and what you have told me so far, I think the reason that you have been unable to pin a diagnosis down and define your symptoms accordingly is because you may have experienced some form of late-onset post-traumatic stress disorder.'

I was intrigued.

'When you were attacked as a child, your mind dealt with it by splitting from your body, and you relived that memory, that whole incidence, twenty-three years later and you split again,' she continued. 'And then, three years later, you split to being fifteen again, at a time when feelings of stability and safety had disappeared, and then . . .' She paused. 'You said earlier that the cause of all of this splitting was stress?'

'Stress?' I was starting to see where she was going with this.

'So maybe what's been happening to your mind is that it has found its own unique way of dealing with the stress of trauma, and any added stress from life or people in your life has caused a pressure so great it's resulted in disorder. It doesn't matter what type essentially because each diagnosis is framed by disorder.'

'I mean, yeah, that makes sense . . . disorder literally means lack of order.' I stopped and digested what Maria had said. It was beginning to make sense to me. 'Lack of order in my mind.' I suddenly saw all these words for disorder: confusion, disturbance, a mess; as Teen Nay would say, a majorly mentally bogus smegfest. It was falling into place. 'Stress.' I uttered the word, such a harmless word, six letters, so small and yet so powerfully harmful.

Stress, the reason my brain had lost the plot and started to perform some form of mentacide, as Teen Nay would say.

'Well, stress can cause physical problems: heart attacks,

strokes, et cetera. If it affects your physical health, why not the mind?' Maria reasoned.

'So why don't people take it as seriously when it's your mental health? Why the shame, the taboo?'

'The debate rages on with that one.' Maria gave a small smile. 'But the question now is what can you, if anything, do about it so that it doesn't happen again?'

'Well . . .' I thought for a moment, and then remembered my newly adopted theory that the answer to my problem was in the problem itself.

'Well, if it is post-traumatic stress disorder, then there's not much I can do about the trauma, and right now it's the "post" part, but I can do something about the stress and the disorderly conduct in my mind.'

'Okay.'

'Well, I first need to understand what post-traumatic stress disorder is exactly and then figure out what I can do to counteract the effects of it, if I can.'

Maria explained to me that post-traumatic stress disorder could be seen as a mental illness caused by extreme trauma. The symptoms could range from depression to flashbacks. The flashbacks could manifest in the form of vivid and distressing nightmares or the unexpected onslaught of painful memories so powerful that a person can actually feel like they are going through the traumatic event again. More often than not the mind gets confused (that'll be the disorderly conduct then) and separates itself from the memory in order to make sense of it. Sometimes, this can manifest as splitting, which if not understood causes further distress, which in turn affects a person's whole life.

I totally got it; mine had been affected because I hadn't understood what was going on. I had no positive way to deal with the flashbacks and the consequent splitting and this pushed me further into crisis.

Maria explained that when a person suffers from post-traumatic stress disorder, they tend to stay away from close emotional relationships with their family and friends. They find difficulty in expressing themselves in these relationships and this frustration can cause anger and grief, which in turn affects their behaviour. This again explained my relationship breakdowns with those close to me, especially my sister, Eve and my friends.

'There is always a sense of being constantly under threat, seeing danger everywhere, even when there isn't any, and this causes paranoia,' Maria added.

'I never felt truly safe around others,' I confessed. 'I used to take razor blades on dates with me and sleep with a bat under my bed.'

'Well, talking of sleep, when you have post-traumatic stress disorder, you can sleep all the time and then not sleep for days. You have trouble concentrating.'

'That explains why I struggled with the work load from university.'

'Yes, in order to cope you become detached, removed from a life that plays out like a movie where you are the spectator, watching yourself, numb to your needs.'

'This started to happen with my holistic therapy business, especially when I was teaching others how to heal. I wasn't a part of what was happening in those classrooms, so it wasn't real to me.' This was all starting to make sense.

'In the end,' Maria continued, 'because of the sheer stress, a person can end up self-medicating a lot, anything from alcohol or drugs to prescription drugs. They have low impulse control and struggle to remain grounded.'

This explained the weed and the cocaine and the Keith Richards lifestyle. I mean, a rolling stone gathers no moss, but wow, not even a bit of soil? As I moved through my life I hadn't taken responsibility for my drug taking, blaming others instead.

'When it reaches this point, you find yourself trapped in a cycle where you are doing things to yourself that you know you shouldn't be doing, only you can't help yourself, even though it's harming you and then, if it gets really bad, you end up wanting to kill yourself.'

'That would explain the suicidal tendencies, then?' I asked.

'Or kill other people.'

'That would explain my violent thoughts.'

'Or get someone to kill you,' she added.

'Well, I didn't quite get there, but may have pissed someone off enough along the way at some point in time if I had carried on,' I joked.

'Which is not because you want to die as such,' Maria continued. 'It's usually because you can no longer live with the pain.'

I sat in silence, absorbing everything she had told me. It was like someone had finally given me a manual for my disordered mind and the key points of the content were spelled clearly, concisely and in order.

'I think I understand this more,' I told Maria. 'Every time I tried to break free, establish my own identity, I was pushed back and then I would split.' I thought back to when I was young. 'I was a precocious child; I liked attention. If there was a room full of people, I wanted their eyes on me. I would perform, sing songs and dance. And then he attacked me, abused me; like he wanted to possess me, have what I had. And then when I was a teenager, my stepdad paid for me to go to dance classes, and my confidence grew again. I was in productions and plays, I went to auditions . . .' I could feel myself welling up. 'And then all of that stopped when he left and my friends were sexually assaulted in school and my mum's life was threatened, and well, then I tried to commit suicide because I couldn't control what was happening. As much as I told myself that I hated her, my mum was really the only stability I knew.'

'What happened after that?' Maria asked gently.

'Well, I blamed myself for what had happened to my friends. I thought it was somehow my fault. We were never the same after that; they had been my safety net and that was taken away. I did so many things to try and keep us together, but in the end we drifted apart.'

A single tear fell and rolled down my cheek. I wiped it away. 'Do you know how many women I have known in my short lifetime that have been raped or sexually abused? Too many. Far, far too many.'

'What happened after you tried to take your own life, Naomi?' she asked carefully.

'Well, I lived with Art, but it didn't work out. My stepmum Marlene had left, disappeared, didn't even say goodbye.'

'How did that make you feel?'

'At the time, I was shocked, stunned even, but didn't really process it, you know? I think I split again, and then when I went to Greece, I realized I was angry with her for leaving. I felt abandoned; she had been part of me growing up. She was part of me trying to find my identity. Growing up, I felt like she had accepted me more.'

'And then?'

It was all clicking into place.

'Well, then I, you know, had Leo and set up my own business and became a teacher. I started to perform again. Once more, I had a stage; people would listen to me, and come back again and again to be taught by me. I was carving out a niche, finding my own identity.'

'And then what happened?'

'Well, I was about to set up my own school and then, well, my world came crashing down again. In her drunken state, Eve told me she didn't know whether Art was my real dad and that my father could possibly be another man.'

The tears spilled thick and fast. Maria leaned forward and passed me a box of tissues.

'Again,' I sobbed through my tears, 'my identity fragmented. It was attached to my father, to his name, to his family, the one constant in my world. And then he became unreliable because of stuff he was going through, which made me question whether I really was his, made me question whether I really mattered, so I split again.'

'Made you question your place in this world? Who you were?'

'Yeah.' I looked Maria in the eye. 'God, I have never really known myself, never really known who I truly am, or even what I am capable of. Every time I have tried, from when I was a little girl, someone or something has always come in and blown me off track, knocked me down, and I've laid there feeling like I can't get up again and the only way I can cope is to split.'

'But you cope. You have coped,' she reassured me. 'Sometimes when you get knocked down and you feel you can't get up again, you need help. You need someone or something to help you get up and keep going.'

'Even splitting?'

Maria nodded.

I wasn't convinced. 'But for most of my life, it's been drugs.'

'What about Leo?'

'Well, that goes without saying – of course Leo. I mean, I often think I wouldn't be here today if it wasn't for him. When I was suicidal through the breakdown, it was the thought of him that stopped me from pressing the razor blades into my flesh.'

The room fell silent. I took a deep breath and wiped the fresh tears.

'Oh gosh,' I sobbed. 'What if he wasn't here? I'd be dead by now.'

'But he is here,' she said softly. 'And you're still here, and that's all that matters right now. But what about you? Or even the child or teen within you? Haven't they helped you? Haven't they lifted you back up when you've been knocked down and felt you couldn't go on?'

I thought about this for a moment. 'Yeah, I suppose they have.'

'Not *they*. You! They were you, you are them, so bottom line, it has been you that has kept you going; it has been you all along who has known who you truly are and what you are truly capable of because it has been you who has picked yourself up and carried on.'

It took a minute for it to sink in, but when it did I finally understood what she was saying. It *was* me. I had survived. I was still alive, I was still breathing and eating and sleeping and laughing and crying. I was still living and I was still here for Leo, and it was me that had done it, and that was all that mattered. There was no need for me to dwell on the fact that I'd 'almost' checked out. I needed to concentrate on the fact that I hadn't.

Since I'd come back, after Egypt, the diaries and short stories I'd been writing, Paris and now therapy had all made me realize that I'd been living most of my life with The Voice.

'The voice?' Maria asked me during one particular breakthrough therapy session.

I nodded. 'Yeah, and just to make sure, I went around to all of my female friends, and some of them have never experienced any form of mental illness, but they all said yes.'

'Yes to what, Naomi?'

'To having a voice. I mean, I know it's taboo, no one wants to talk about the voices in your head but . . .' I stopped and when Maria didn't say anything, I added, 'I bloody well am going to now, I need to.'

'Go on,' she encouraged.

'I need to expose the voice in my head that I have had for as long as I can remember, telling me time and time again that I am not good enough, you know? It tells me that I can't do it, that I won't be able to do it, and if I try, I will fail. It tells me I am not pretty enough, tall enough, slim enough or talented enough. It tells me that I am weak when I most need strength; it tells me I am a fool when I seek wisdom; it tells me I am undeserving when I want love.' I could feel a deep well of emotion rising to the surface. I took a deep breath. 'It's pushed me into a fearful place, it's attacked me at my most vulnerable and it's been so unforgiving when I have made mistakes.'

My body began to throb with the force of this emotion. I paused for a moment and thought about all of the women who had said pretty much the same thing to me about The Voice. 'It's so powerful,' I added as the tears spilled over.

Maria played out the familiar and comforting act of passing me the box of tissues. I took one, blew my nose loudly and smiled.

'Thank you.'

'Powerful how, Naomi?' She wanted me to continue talking.

'Well, I figure that when I was born, I had a space around me and this space was empty, and over the years this space has just got filled up with stuff.'

'Stuff?'

'Yeah, just stuff, you know, from my parents, friends, society, my environment . . .' I reeled off a list. 'But at some point my space started to get filled up with crap, horrible stuff that told me I was wrong, and this sense of wrongness has followed me into adulthood.'

I looked down at the green top I was wearing and pulled on it. 'I had the wrong clothes – they were not expensive enough. I had the wrong hair type – it wasn't straight, blonde, curly or soft enough. I had the wrong body – my breasts were too small or my thighs too big. I didn't speak properly or I couldn't write in the correct way. I was the wrong colour, gender, class or culture. I wasn't rich enough, smart enough, clever enough . . .' I took another deep breath and thought about the magazines and television Teen Nay had experienced in my future and how they had made her feel.

'You know what as well? I have also realized that television has fed my space, books have fed my space, pictures from magazines and newspapers have fed my space.'

I started to cry again. 'Strangers that hurt me, family members that bullied me. Bosses that didn't recognize my work, boyfriends that belittled me. Friends that talked about me. It's all fed this space around me.'

'What has this got to do with The Voice?' Maria asked me softly.

'It's all fertilizer for this bullshit voice; it helps it grow. All this stuff in my space gives The Voice power, and who I am has become so crushed underneath the weight of this stuff that I have broken into pieces, and even if I have tried to find and fix those pieces back together, somehow The Voice has always got in the way.'

'What do you think, if anything, you could do about it?'

'I have to stop it now.'

'The Voice?'

'No, feeding it. I have to watch what stuff I fill my space up with and make sure that it's not stuff that is feeding the voice, making it more powerful.'

'What do you hope that will achieve?'

I stopped and thought about her question for a moment. I had never really thought about what was needed beyond changing the people, places and things in my life that helped The Voice. And then it came to me.

'I suppose when I do, when I eventually get rid of the old stuff and fill my space up with stuff that is good for me, that tells me that I am good enough, well then, maybe I'll find my own voice, the one that comes from me and only wants what is right for me. Yeah.' Smiling, I wiped my wet face with more tissue. 'Maybe my voice will show me who I really am and tell me what I need to live an authentic life, a life with a healed mind.'

'Imagine for a moment if it did – what would it say to you?'

I stopped and closed my eyes and then I could hear it clearly, a voice that was soft and gentle and kind and full of love for me. I listened.

'It would tell me that I am strong and capable and wise, and that I know, deep down underneath all of my stuff, who I am and what I need.'

'What is that?'

I opened my eyes and smiled at Maria. 'I am about to find out.'

15
Letting Go

Many of us spend our whole lives running from feeling
with the mistaken belief that you cannot bear the pain.
But you have already borne the pain.
What you have not done is feel
all you are beyond the pain.

SAINT BARTHOLOMEW

I left Maria's office full of determination to change my life. Now I understood that the amnesia was my mind's way of telling me that the stress had to stop and I wasn't going to ignore it. I needed to continue my own rescuing. I had to listen to Teen Nay and honour what she had experienced and follow through with the changes she had started to make. I didn't want to live a life that prompted the memory loss any longer.

First thing was admitting that starting something important and not finishing it had a negative and debilitating effect on my psyche; I knew I needed to finish my psychology degree once and for all. Not having that sense of completion had contributed to the low self-esteem I had before the amnesia.

I contacted my university to enquire whether it was too late for me to retake my final four exams. They were very accommodating and because of my 'circumstances', were willing to give me one more chance (my very last chance) to resit them. I got to work. It was now July and I had until September to prepare so I pulled out all of my old books and coursework and drew up a study schedule. It seemed that working on the film sets had got me used to the routine of going to bed at a decent hour, getting adequate amounts of sleep, and working all day with breaks.

Surprisingly, this time I found myself enjoying relearning the work, especially abnormal psychology and brain and behaviour. Having now had first-hand knowledge of amnesia, I had a different perspective on the study of memory loss and a new-found respect for the brain.

During this intense period of studying, a woman turned up at my door, introducing herself as Rosalyn, my new mental health social worker. Rosalyn was tall, stood straight-backed, and wore her strawberry blonde hair in a sharp bob. Her black glasses and grey suit added to the oracular cloud surrounding her. She was serious, to the point and she scared me. Teen Nay said she was like my old teacher Mrs O'Shea, who, when you actually sat and listened to her, you realized was a really great teacher who you could learn a lot from. Still, I didn't know Rosalyn so decided I wasn't going to trust her and needed to be careful about what I said.

Intuitively I knew that Rosalyn was one of those women who relied on her instinct as well as her social work knowledge and I knew I wouldn't be able to pull the wool over her eyes. So, in true contradictory style, I decided to pull the veil of illusion over my whole existence instead and peep nervously from behind it like a young Arab girl peering from behind her hijab at the authoritative patriarch.

Rosalyn was supportive of my commitment to retaking my exams and approved of my new routine. But there was one thing – my dark and pungent secret that I couldn't let her find out, no matter what. I was still smoking weed. I wasn't smoking as much as I had done, but nonetheless, I was still experiencing the emotional need to get high. Of course, I knew it didn't fit in with the psychologically healthy life I was envisioning for myself. In the past I had quit on several occasions and abstained for long periods of time, usually when I was at my happiest and most content. But whenever a crisis occurred, one I couldn't cope with, I went straight back to the Mary Jane to suppress the emotion until it manifested in some other way. But I knew a sixteen-year habit wouldn't allow itself to be eradicated so easily. It would go fighting, kicking and screaming. I wanted to quit but how was I going to do it on my own?

I turned to Maria, the one person I knew would listen and not judge me. For the first time in my therapeutic life, I was truly willing to take a long hard look at myself and make the changes necessary to live a 'better' life. I loved having the space, if only for an hour a week, where I could sit and be myself and talk to someone who didn't know me, had no emotional attachment to my life, and only knew what I told her every time I sat in that chair.

'Why does keeping secrets destroy such a huge part of who you are?' I said to her during a particularly hard session.

'Can you elaborate?' Maria asked.

I nodded. 'I've just realized that most of my issues are because of keeping secrets.' I paused and thought about it some more. 'I mean, no matter what is happening to you or around you, you can't tell anybody what is going on, for fear of what will happen to you or those you love.'

'Is this what happened with you?'

'Yes. The men who abused me when I was little told me they would kill my mum and sister if I told anybody what was happening. So I never told.'

'How does this make you feel? Were there other secrets you had to keep?' Maria asked me.

I nodded. 'It makes me feel sad, and angry, but angry where I want to scream it out all over the place.' I thought about Eve. 'Well, the landscape of alcoholism photographs in quite the same way.'

'What do you mean?'

'We wore the facade of the fake, smiling family that was hiding the secret of the illness that was destroying our family from the inside out.'

'Why do you think this is?' Maria asked me gently.

'Well, it's because you're afraid of people getting involved and the secret being found out, but I know now, if I want to live an authentic life, I have to stop with the fear of exposing these damaging secrets and let them out. I am not a child anymore; I am an adult and I feel like I am colluding with my own self-destructive self.'

Maria asked me whether I had any other secrets that I wanted to tell her. I did and told her that in spite of everything, I still had the need to get high. I explained that it calmed the panic, quelled the anxiety, and made me go from not being able to cope to thinking, *Everything happens for a reason; chill out and one day it will all become clear.*

I needed to know whether I could do this naturally without drugs. I needed to know how to think this way without the aid of an illegal substance.

Maria suggested I tell Rosalyn. I burst into tears and covered my face with my hands.

'Naomi, what do you think will happen if you tell?' Maria leaned forward slightly in her chair.

My heart was pounding as I forced myself to look her straight in the eye. 'I think she'll take Leo off me.'

'For smoking weed?' she asked with bemused concern.

'For everything.' Fresh tears rolled down my already soaked cheeks. Even as I said it, I knew it sounded ridiculous, but my fear was genuine.

Maria's question had made me see my situation for what it was: I was a meditating, Jungian, journal-writing pothead, who smoked one or two joints a night outside in the garden when Leo was in bed. I wasn't a hard-core drug addict who had sold all the furniture and was neglecting to feed my child. Maria reassured me that Leo was not at risk and wouldn't be taken off me. The best thing I could do for myself, she said, was to tell Rosalyn that I was still smoking weed.

In that moment I surrendered to the help on offer. And I felt unburdened enough to spend the rest of the session exploring the reasons why I'd started to smoke in the first place.

After my suicide attempt I had gone to live with Art in Liverpool. I was sixteen, in an unfamiliar city, struggling to find a job, friendless and directionless. Then I'd met Angel, a short curly-blonde-haired fifteen-year-old, who lived near my Aunty Mae's house. Angel's mum was good friends with Aunty Mae and I met them both one night while I was there. Angel hadn't finished school and was having serious issues with her mum. Maybe her mum thought I was a good influence, because when I wasn't getting on with Art she let me live with them for a time. When her mum's boyfriend used to stay, we would wait until they were asleep and then Angel and I would sneak out of the living room window and into the bad part of town to flirt with the young drug sellers on the street corner and haggle for a five-pound bag of weed.

For someone who hated drinking, the first bag I was given was 'weed dipped in brandy and then dried at optimum room temperature for a smooth smoke' (the guy was the Donald Trump of Drug Alley and an effective salesman). Smoking my first joint gave me a high I had never experienced before, all warm and fuzzy and sweet, and I spent the next sixteen years looking for that same buzz. Needless to say, I'd never found it.

With Maria's help, I could see, all these years down the line, that our need to engage in faux delinquent behaviour was the only way we both could control our uncertain environment and unstable lives. Missing my family, as dysfunctional as it was, created an emotional void that I was trying to fill with acceptance from my peers. In this case, the drug sellers on the corner and a teen who had issues with her mum.

Now, I wanted – needed – absolution, redemption, forgiveness for being so weak-minded, for turning to drugs when things got too much in life and for not being 'normal' enough to deal with life's ups and downs like everyone else. Telling Rosalyn was akin to being a devout Catholic and waiting to go into confessional to absolve my sins to the hard-nosed priest . . .

To my surprise and great relief, Rosalyn was fantastic. She didn't judge me or scold me. Instead, she admitted she'd thought something was wrong with me and had suspected I'd started to smoke weed again. She pulled out her diary and wrote down a number for the local substance misuse service, ripping out the page for me. She said she would refer me to a key worker so that I could go on their twelve-step programme and get the help I needed.

I had never felt so relieved. It seemed as if a big weight had been lifted and I could at long last let go of all the years of taking drugs. To finally release the constant battle of contradiction felt redemptive. Strangely, even more so because Rosalyn was someone who didn't know me but was on my side. She was here to offer me temporary support. And when she assured me that the last thing she was going to do was take my child off me, I felt so much relief I hugged her.

Several days later, a woman from the twelve-step programme called Anna contacted me and arranged for me to go and meet her the following week. I was nervous and even slightly sceptical, but I forced myself to go.

Anna was a small, round, comfortably built, pink-cheeked woman with masses of buttery curls that sprang from all over her head, reminding me of the bunches of spiralled ribbon you find on birthday presents. She had a strong Bolton accent and gave a slight giggle after every sentence as if exchanging the word 'the' for the letter T was a dialectic joke I wasn't privy to.

After our first meeting I had it figured out: Anna was a genuinely happy person. She didn't put it on; it wasn't an act. She had a sunny disposition, which living in Manchester (with all the rain) was rare. I was usually wary of happy people; I didn't trust them. I believed it took way too much energy to be consistently happy and, somewhere underneath it all, was a miserable wretch just waiting for the right opportunity to pounce up and devour you with years of suppressed anger and latent hostility. But Anna challenged that belief and the greatest thing was her verve for life was in no way patronizing because I got this sense that she knew exactly what I was going through. While I couldn't imagine Anna ever stealing your flat-screen TV so she could score that night, I knew the look. It was an empathic understanding mixed with a peaceful smile and a quiet joy. I had never seen this in myself. I was seeing it in Anna and I wanted to not only know it, but own it.

She took me through the services provided and how best they could help me. I thought we were going to have to explore the reasons I had started smoking weed in the first place, as I had done with Maria, and how it had led to speed, LSD, ecstasy and cocaine. But as much as my drug-taking past mattered, she kept bringing the conversation to the here and now and what we could do to stop me from smoking. The need to snort coke or drop a bomb of speed wasn't strong anymore, but the first thing I had to do, she instructed me, was to go home and carry on smoking and keep to my usual routine of a joint or two a night. Except this time, I needed to write down exactly when I was starting to want one and how I felt before I did. Then I was to write down how I felt while stoned and then write down how I felt and what I thought once it had worn off.

I did this for several days and then began to see a pattern. The 'negative-internal-dialogue-creates-anxiety-and-results-in-panic' pattern. It would hit at a certain time in the day – around four p.m. – and I would start to grow inexplicably anxious. That anxiety would sit like a small ball of wool at the bottom of my stomach, and by the time Leo was in bed, I would be so tense from trying to stop that ball unravelling that I would start to panic and need something to make it go away. Trying to see where the ball came from filled me with a terrible dread and the only thing that had the power to push it down as far as it would go was weed. For the time the weed lasted, I felt calm and relaxed, and the fear dissipated. As it began to wear off the panic would come back again and I would smoke another. And so the cycle went.

After about two weeks of writing this down, I realized I wasn't actually dealing with the issue that made me start in the first place. I was just dumbing it down, tranquillizing it until it stopped. I needed to address it head-on. But this was easier said than done, so eventually, after a couple of nights of observing my feelings before going through the ritual of smoking and not understanding the anxiety, I turned to Teen Nay, who was watching quietly from her room in the house.

Me: *What shall I do? I am a nervous wreck.*
Her: *Remember when things were tense at home or we felt stressed with school?*
Me: *Yeah.*
Her: *What did we do?*
Me: *Errr . . .*
Her: *We went for a walk.*

It was a simple thing but the thought was surprising to me because it had not entered my head before. Exercise had always been a way to lose weight or keep healthy, never to deal with my emotions.

Her: *Go for a walk, dude! Oh, and one more thing, Adult Naomi, I know it's all slush puppies, but . . . thank you and . . . I kinda love you.*
Me: *I kinda love you too, Teen Nay, and, no, thank you.*

So, I started walking. An hour or so after Leo had fallen asleep, I would leave the house and walk up and down my street, sometimes thinking about Teen Nay, sometimes listening to music, but most importantly, not thinking about getting high. The first few times I smoked after walking, but felt good because I had delayed the smoking so was therefore smoking less. I also noticed the feelings of anxiety and nervous tension were slowly subsiding and, after a power walk, I felt exhilarated, powerful. My head was clearer and one night the source of the negative thoughts became apparent.

It was all about feeling safe. The key to being at ease once I was on my own was to create feelings of safety and stability, which in turn made me feel secure. Moving home so much as a child, the expectation of abuse during the night, the lack of reliable emotional attachments, all created a constant underlying tension that translated as the inability to feel safe. I'd never felt truly secure.

This 'exercise epiphany' hinted at a life where I was able to control the negative emotion and find a way to create these elusive feelings of natural well-being.

Without getting high! Bonus!

I shared this with Anna, and the steps after this encouraged me to find different things to do, other than walking, to make me feel just as good. Aside from writing, I found knitting kept my fingers occupied and baking cakes for Leo, Katie and her brood was therapeutic. Delivering the cakes in the evening got me out of the house and the smiles on her children's faces when they bit into my chocolate fudge brownies contributed to a slow-growing self-esteem. I didn't have to find things I liked about myself; I just needed to remember what was already great about me. Life was becoming an earnest search for serotonin-inducing activities.

And then I was sent to a place called Oddfellows House, a small red-bricked building with a car park at the back, that was used by the substance misuse service as a meeting place for what I liked to call my Fellow Followers of Oddity and where we all tried to figure our way out of a whole heap of pain. These followers were ex-heroin addicts, crack-smokers, and amphetamine-takers, with a couple of alcoholics thrown in for good measure. Most were men, a couple were women, and every Friday morning we ate toast, drank tea, and discussed what it was like coming off our particular drug of choice and what we were doing to ensure we wouldn't go back to it. Some part of the morning involved us sitting around a large table, having acupuncture needles stuck in our ears (to help with the craving). We looked like some form of hybrid version of metal-eared aliens, wide-eyed, and toothless (the older drug addicts), trying to figure out if the funny tingling in our ears was really trapped energy releasing itself or just wax dislodging. After this there was the option of a free massage or reiki, which involves someone placing their hands on you to transfer healing energy into your body.

Some Fridays, I would partake in the conversations; other times I would take my university revision and listen to others talk while I read about the mind and behaviour.

Jimmy joined the sessions about three weeks after I started. He didn't say much at first so I didn't take much notice of him. He was a tall, stooping-through-the-door type of man, skinny and long. He had shaved light blond hair, a sallow complexion, and when he spoke his two missing front teeth gave him a slight lisp.

I noticed him the day that a few of us were all sitting around the table in silence, while the group leader (I nicknamed him Acupuncture Guy) walked slowly from one of us to the next, pulling the small copper needles out of our ears. The ambience in the room was very relaxed, chilled to the point of a narcoleptic atmosphere, with soft music playing in the background, and my brain felt like it wanted to curl up and fall asleep. One of the men, Joe, a recovering alcoholic, broke the silence. He started talking about pain – the pain he felt from the needles and the pain he felt now he wasn't drinking.

'It's like there, you know?' He looked at us all sitting around the table. 'And I, like, don't know what to do with it. I wanna let it out, but I don't know how. Without it . . . you know, like, really hurting. Without it killing me.'

We all nodded; we all understood what he was talking about. Pain and what to do with it, how to express it, how to cope with it, how to deal with it.

The mood was serious and then Jimmy piped up. Shaking

his head, he said in a thick Lancashire accent, 'I know what ya mean, mate; it's like plaiting snot in fog.'

I was the first to burst into a loud laugh. He looked at me, puzzled for a moment, and then a smile curled from the corner of his mouth and he started to chuckle.

Joe began to laugh too and then everyone followed and the room was filled with laughter.

Even Acupuncture Guy's broad shoulders moved up and down in time to his silent laughter.

Once we calmed down, Acupuncture Guy proceeded to tell us about organized group walks up in the hills of the Pennines that we could go on.

But it had me thinking about emotional pain. We all laughed, but really, why did we find it so difficult to deal with? I had pushed out a 9lb 9 baby, with no drugs. My physical pain threshold was high, so why wasn't it the same for my emotional pain?

It was then that I looked individually at each and every one of the men and women sitting around the table. We were all so different – in age, in sex, in colour even – but we all felt a common bond: our struggle with pain, and how to manage the energy of hurt before it became really painful, before the energy moved and threatened to destroy you.

It was at that moment that I realized that the 'e' in emotion was energy and the 'motion' was the movement of that energy. If it hurt, my natural reaction was to push it out; like whenever I got a splinter as a child, adults always told me to leave it because eventually my body would gather all the necessary resources to push it out. But with emotion, something would have happened at some point in our lives that told us to resist the movement and instead, do the opposite, and pull back. That's when we got scared, anxious, and panicked because we didn't know what to do with it. So we pulled it back and pushed it down, tried to force it back to where it came from: its point of origin. Except the force of the energy was so powerful, so strong, that once it had begun to move, no force within us was strong enough to hold it down forever.

As I watched all of us sitting around the table, I realized that whether it was an attack, a death, rape, beatings, abuse or torture, they all led to one thought, one negative belief about ourselves, pushed into a space where it had no choice but to fold back on itself and double over, causing a pressure which eventually had to move: e-motion, energy in motion. Our resistance against this movement caused the pain and we reached for something – a spliff, a pipe, a drink, a needle – to push it back down where it would fold again. A continuous pile-on, thought over thought, feeling over feeling, piling on, pushing down. Ours was a fight, a battle of resistance; our drug of choice was the weapon.

Oddfellows House was for the battle-worn, the ones who had decided the fight was no longer right for them. Something in us had awoken to the idea that we could find a way, find some answer to the pain. That maybe moving towards it and through it and letting it out would somehow be better for us than moving against it and away from it and keeping it in. It was, after all, energy, and when we reached that point, the beginning before that energy moved and became emotion, there was something in us, buried deep inside of us, that could actually deal with the pain.

We at Oddfellows House were at odds with our true selves,

with that true voice, the part of us that could deal with living a truthful life. This was the voice Teen Nay had sought in Egypt, the source of my true self, the point of origin of my own energy. She had needed to find it and for me to see it so that I understood my own validity in this life, my own purpose. Who I am before the pain, what happens to me going through the pain but, more importantly, who I become after the pain.

Later, Jimmy joined me in the reading room, where the day's newspapers were laid out, and where I usually went to study. After a while, he put his paper down. I glanced up and saw that he was rubbing his hand; it was slightly red. He noticed me watching him and I gave him a friendly smile.

'I dint mean to make ya laff, ya know. T'was all serious, like, an' I go an' be the bloody joker.'

'Naaa, it's okay. Sometimes we could all do with a good laugh,' I reassured him.

He rubbed his hand again.

'Did you hurt your hand?' I assumed he'd hurt it searching for a viable vein to take his daily requirements of brown.

'Me kid bit me.' His face lit up.

'What? Oh, wow! Bit of a naughty one, then?' Why was he happy about it?

He shook his head and laughed. 'Na. It's me own fault. I was teasin 'im rite bout avin skid marks in't boxes (boxer shorts), an' then he bit me, an' I ses what ya do that for? I can see ya teef print on me, an' he ses, that's ya kid mark.'

I don't know why I found this guy hilarious, but I did and I creased up laughing again. Jimmy chuckled along with me and then we proceeded to talk about the wonders of being a single parent. He was the proud parent of an eight-year-old girl and a six-year-old joker of a son. Their mother, a heroin addict herself, had run away to Folkestone with his friend. Jimmy's children were in foster care, but he and his mother had managed to get temporary custody of them, one of the conditions being that he cleaned himself up and got off heroin for good, which was why he was at Oddfellows House. By the time we had finished chatting I was convinced he had not yet met his calling as a stand-up comedian. He was hilarious and completely oblivious to it.

On my way home, I continued my thoughts about pain. Jimmy had spent most of his life using opiates to hide from his. But when he knew he was the only one left there for his children, he had finally decided the pain of losing them would be far greater than the pain he was feeling now.

Pale white horse in comparison.

Still, horsemen of the apocalypse aside, I realized Jimmy and I were truly no different; we had different lives, and had experienced different storms, but we were both on the same search. Both he and I needed to change and we were both at Oddfellows House because the pain of staying the same was greater than the pain of changing.

With all of these thoughts swimming around my head, when I got home, I decided to do as much research as I could about pain. I found an infinite amount of information but one thing that made me stop in my tracks was a video clip I found of the recorded sound of a plant growing from a seed through the soil to reach the air above it. The recording sounded like screaming. The growth for the plant, the pushing against the soil into the air and towards the sun above it where it could blossom, was painful. That pain was caused by nothing other than resistance, pushing against something as strong and powerful as the earth, and yet the small seedling found a way.

I thought about how, even after all Jimmy and I had been through, we still managed to laugh, still managed to find humour in everyday life. And then it came to me: my pain was transient; it didn't last. It always had a beginning, and a middle, and there was always an end. I realized that I could use this knowledge as a force to propel me through the experience of the pain, to allow it to come out instead of me pushing it down. If I did, then maybe one day I would find myself on the other side of it.

Jimmy and I were the seeds, the growing flowers; events meant that we were growing in different ways, but growing nonetheless, only to reach the same place. Who we truly were and where we belonged under the sun.

Growing up around smokers and drinkers was a normal part of everyday life, but it meant that health was never at the forefront of my mind. The only exercise I ever did was at school and even then I tried everything to get out of P.E. by regularly sticking my fingers down my throat and telling Mrs Dixon of Dock Green (she was tall and looked like a policeman) that I had my period four weeks a month. Teen Nay reminded me of this in one of her diary entries when she had started to exercise. This made me think about health and the fact that you could find the word 'heal' in it. I soon realized after the amnesia that dealing with my mental health meant at some point dealing with my physical health. Especially my brain, which of course was in control of everything my body did.

For the first time in my life 'shopping for personal trainers' didn't mean searching for tailor-made Adidas to fit my huge size nine feet. No, instead it meant I found Gary, 'fitness expert to the stars', on the Internet. He was tall and fair, and he had the most intense blue eyes and a refreshingly no-nonsense attitude to health, coupled with a kind and understanding nature. He was an ex-athlete and a fantastic trainer. I had not yet met anyone who had quit smoking weed and actually put weight on, but I had managed it, so Gary sent me to a nutritionist and came up with a healthy eating and exercise plan. I was apparently severely dehydrated and had very little lung capacity, which along with the excess weight were temporary things that could be fixed, and he told me that if I put in the commitment, time and energy, then my health goals could be achieved.

Throughout our time in the gym, Gary also became somewhat of a therapist and I found myself telling him how I was quitting smoking and that I was in therapy to work out my issues. More importantly, I told him about losing my memory and being fifteen years of age again, how my life had turned out to be a colossal disappointment to Teen Nay and that I needed to keep the promise I had made to change my life. He listened intently and then assured me he would do anything he could in his power to help me keep that promise.

During one session, about a month into the training, he said something to me that was so simple but which changed the way I saw my mind and how it worked. Working out that particular morning was a struggle and, while boxing the punchbag, I burst into tears. I was fed up and tired of going to bed every night on my own. I was missing male company and after the break-up with French Dude was sad that I had experienced another unsuccessful relationship. I ended up telling Gary how I felt. I told him about the relationship pattern that was no longer working for me (prince + princess + rescue = Disney) and that I wasn't sure if I knew how to relate to men any other way. He listened while instructing me to continue with my sit-ups and then stopped me.

'Every time you talk to yourself in a negative way or criticize yourself—' he started.

'I know, I know,' I said rolling my eyes.

'No, Naomi, you don't.' He looked at me intently. 'You increase your stress hormones. Stress hormones tell your body there is danger, and then your body craves rich and sugary foods for a quick burst of energy.'

'To escape the danger?' I had an idea where he was going with this.

'Yes. Then your body produces a hormone called ghrelin to defend itself from stress, anxiety or depression—'

'Let me guess,' I interrupted, 'this makes me want more sugar?'

'Actually, it makes you hungrier; it's your hunger hormone.'

This was all brand new to me. 'So . . . ?' I hoped he had the answer.

'So if you stop beating yourself up for every mistake you make and talk to yourself with respect, this will produce oxytocin and serotonin, your feel-good hormones, and these will help your brain deal with stress and, in turn, decrease your hunger and cravings.'

'Okay.' I was listening hard now.

'And, of course, meditation or exercise produces those hormones as well. They are the most powerful stress relievers and effective antidepressants – way, way better than drugs.' He looked at me proudly, as if he had just given me the answer to the meaning of life itself.

'Okay and what's this got to do with my ex-boyfriends?'

'Haven't the foggiest. Don't ask me about relationships; I'm still figuring out why I'm getting married.'

He picked up the leather boxing gloves and tossed them over to me.

'Well, you said some of them smoked, right? Or drank excessively or took drugs?' Gary asked.

'Yeah, I've scraped the bottom of the broken barrel with some of my choices in boyfriends,' I said, putting the gloves back on.

'So, maybe if you took care of yourself a bit more and learned how to love being healthy, then maybe you'll meet a man who does also, and if he does, then he'd be naturally happier, and in turn you would be too. Happy people are infectious.' He grinned and held on to the punchbag.

I thought for a moment, *Learn to love being healthy.* I knew people had been doing it for hundreds of years, but it was a completely new concept to me.

'Exercise regularly, whether it's a twenty-minute walk to the shop or a swim in your local pool and, well, watch: things will start to change, especially your mind.' He pulled the punchbag over to me.

And in that moment, I decided that the negative self-talk just had to stop. I wasn't going to beat myself up anymore.

Instead, as I punched the bag, I thought about the simple concept of learning to love being healthy. It was a light-bulb moment for me and it lit up my healing mind.

I passed my final exams with flying colours and graduated with first-class honours. I finished my twelve steps and left Anna proud that I had completed the programme. I was ready to see what a life without drugs was like. Rosalyn noticed the positive changes in me and started to talk about discharging me, how I no longer needed support from social services. And I was making progress with Maria, examining my relationship with myself, the ways in which I was turning it from a dysfunctional into a healthy one. We spoke at length about my female relationships, particularly with Eve and Simone, and ways in which I could positively work through my feelings, reconciling past events with the present, finding healing in the work I was doing now.

Life could be lived if I took small steps, one day at a time: little goals to focus on and small rewards if they were achieved. This was my existence and it was all I felt like I could manage.

I began to believe that if I remained like this, then things would get better and eventually I would become the person Teen Nay knew I could be.

The true me.

And then, one day, I received a phone call that changed everything.

Again.

16

Forgiveness

*Forgiveness is the fragrance
that the violet sheds
on the heel
that has crushed it.*

Mark Twain

It was a mid-October day and Leo was at Simone's for the weekend. Although I still wasn't speaking to her, I didn't want to stop them seeing each other. I had decided to use the time to catch up on the housework and was elbow-deep in soapy water washing the dishes when Leo called me.

'Hiya, mate,' I answered. 'Are you okay?'

'Yeah.'

'What are you up to?'

'Simone's moving to Dubai,' he blurted out.

'What?'

'Yeah, she said that she's moving to the Middle East. To work in a school. And I can go and visit her anytime I want.'

'Oh, wow.' I was so shocked I hardly knew what I was saying. 'Um, that's so cool.'

'Yeah.' He seemed happy.

'When is she leaving?'

'Errr, hang on.' I heard a muffled sound from the phone. 'She said next week.'

I almost dropped the phone. 'Really?' I strained my throat, trying to hide the lump forming.

'Yeah.'

'That's great, isn't it, mate?' I didn't know what else to say other than to focus on how he felt about it.

'I can't wait to go.'

'What are you doing now?' I changed the subject.

'I'm having my dinner and then I'm gonna go and play at Tom's house.'

'Cool. Well, I'll see you when you get home tomorrow.'

'Okay, Mum. Love you, bye.'

'Bye, son, love you too,' I whispered.

I stared into the 'soft as your face' bubbles floating across the murky dishwater, three thoughts hop-stepping my emotions into a frenzy: *I can't believe she's leaving me, I can't believe she's going so far,* and *How dare she leave Eve here alone in Manchester, with no other next of kin but me.* The overwhelming sense of abandonment produced an anger that threatened to swallow me up and I wanted to smash every dish in the sink. This wasn't what was supposed to happen. In my mind, it was going to play out like the Sandra Bullock movie where she ends up in rehab, eventually reconciling her addiction and healing the damage she has caused. Eve was going to play Sandra's character and I was going to receive a phone call from her therapist saying she wanted to have family therapy with me and Simone and we would get to air all our grievances and heal some of the wounds caused by her alcoholism and destructive behaviour.

Simone's decision to move abroad was a big wake-up call. That Hollywood Happy Ending was never going to happen. I felt like that helpless teenager again, whose sister had gone to Malta, leaving me to deal with Eve and our fractured relationship. Over the past few months, keeping my distance from them both had given me some sense of power or control over the situation. And now, within a heartbeat, that power had been taken away. Although I wasn't speaking to her, I had thought at some point that things would eventually go back to normal. Now I wondered whether they ever would.

A couple of days later I received an email from my sister explaining why she was going and that she loved me and would miss me, and because I was angry, I wrote back wishing her well, remaining resolute in my conviction that not speaking to her would be the best thing for me. But it seemed like a more powerful force was at work as the Internet crashed and the message wouldn't go, so instead I sat with Maria, and cried to her about how abandoned and angry I felt being left with the 'sick' mother and how I felt as though I had no choice but to be there for her if she needed me. All sorts of extreme scenarios were crowding my mind. If Eve was sober now, I didn't trust that she was going to stay that way for any positive amount of time. I envisioned her wandering the streets drunk and hurt like the last time I saw her and me being the only person left to deal with that. I didn't want it. I did not want that to be my reality, but at the same time, felt such an immense guilt for not wanting to be there for my mother, even though the situation was so potentially destructive to me.

In her calm and reassuring way, Maria helped me deconstruct my thoughts, to see my sister and my mother as separate entities and not this malevolent force that had always been against me since childhood, against me growing into the person I had always wanted to be. I also had – for the first time – to sincerely try and deal with, and work past, my feelings of envy towards Simone, especially her ability to just pick up and leave and travel the world or work somewhere new and exciting. Where I was left to deal with an unknown future.

Why did she always seem to have it so easy? Opportunities just seemed to fall into her lap and present her with amazing adventures. She had good credit, she held down a secure job, she had a pension, and a great group of friends that loved her for being her, and now she was going to work in a glamorous city and leave me to fend for myself.

The amount of negative emotion entangled in these beliefs was going to take more than one therapy session to unravel. However, Maria helped me begin to see Simone for the human being she was, the compassionate woman and daughter who just wanted to help her mother as best she could and provide her with the help and support to get sober. She wasn't just a sister, there for me to rely on in times of need, or an aunty to take care of her nephew when I needed a break. She was her own person, with her own fears and hopes and dreams, and she was trying her best, just as much as any other person, given the emotional tools she had accumulated in life.

Maria allowed me to see that being a source of support and watching what I had been through all of her life must have taken its toll on Simone, providing her with no small degree of guilt at being the sister who didn't experience it, but witnessed it nonetheless. For so long, I had been the one telling everybody my siblings hadn't understood my upbringing because they hadn't experienced the mother I'd had. They'd got the mother that played with them, baked cakes with them, treated them like children, and allowed them to enjoy their youth. This, in my opinion, hadn't been my experience, and I had come to the conclusion that it was difficult – almost impossible – for them to reconcile such a marked difference in our experiences. I had always felt like the odd one out, the rejected child who got blamed for everything while they hadn't even known or seen that side of my mother. That is, all of them except Simone. A sister who, for a long time, had dealt with the effects of that adversity and never really complained and now she, in her love for the mother she had, was trying her best to help and heal her own experience of the past.

I'd never really thought about my sister's side of things until Maria pointed this entire truth out to me. I left her room that day feeling at peace with my sister leaving, even though I knew I was heading for an intense period of grieving because we were finally coming to the end of an era I had wanted to end for so long. Eve, my sister and I had been struggling to let go of a pattern for so many years – the alcoholic co-dependant triangle. This was her bid for independence and leaving was a testament to her needing that as much as it was a reflection of me needing to work things out on my own. I had to come to terms with the fact that it wasn't only men I turned to, looking for rescue when I was in crisis, but my sister too, and I had to let go of her as well as the men. When I left my session with Maria, I realized that I was about to get what I had asked for. It just hadn't come the way I'd expected it to.

Still, I didn't know what to say to Simone and found myself unable to pick up the phone. It had been eight months since I had heard her voice. But luckily she phoned me the night before she left for Dubai and our conversation confirmed everything that had come to light with Maria.

'Hiya, babe,' she said softly.

'Hi, Sim.' I couldn't hide the sadness from my voice.

'Are you okay?'

'Yeah.' No, I wasn't, and as much as I wanted to be happy for her, I needed to be honest and voice my unhappiness. 'No, I'm not, Simone, but I will be.'

'I know, girl. I just need to go, Naomi.' Her voice wavered. 'I need a break, Nay. I just wanted to go anywhere, a holiday cruise, just two weeks in a tropical paradise, anywhere where I could just look after me and focus on me for a while. You know, work out what I want for myself. And then this job came up and I got an interview and it's my chance to get away, you know?'

'Yeah.' I thought back to Egypt and Teen Nay's driving need to get away and find out who she, who I really was. I understood.

'Not that there is anything wrong, per se, with the old me.' She laughed. 'You know, in essence, I am still the same person. Dizzy, loving, loud, opinionated!'

I smiled and wiped my tears.

'But I still care; I'm still compassionate and empathetic, although I can be a gob shite.' I burst out laughing at this. 'And I know I can be indecisive, moody, and honest . . . sometimes too honest.' She laughed.

'Yeah,' I agreed, but it was also one thing I loved about her; you always needed one person in your life who wasn't afraid to be honest with you and that person for me was Simone.

'But you're going.' More tears started to form.

'I know, hun, but when I was driving back from dropping my friends at the airport early one morning I was overwhelmed with panic, trying to figure out how I would get the money together to go on a break somewhere on the other side of the world. I prayed for God to please give me a sign. I started the car and the radio came on and that song came on, you know?' And she started singing the Crystal Waters song about leaving her job, her car and home and going to a destination unknown, in a high-pitched, off-key voice.

I continued to laugh. I knew the song, so I sang along as if the *X Factor* judges themselves were watching me. She joined in, and we both sang the whole song together down the phone to each other and then creased up laughing. It reminded me of when we were little and we'd sit in the bathroom (we thought the acoustics made us sound like Whitney Houston) and belt out songs. The tears stopped and I realized wherever she went in the world, we would always have a true unbreakable sisterly bond that, no matter how much time had passed or how much distance between us, would always be there.

'Babe, it's just that I've been supporting you from a young age, and I feel like I need to do something for myself now. We've fought like cats and dogs and annoyed each other

forever, but I always have and always will love you throughout our ups and downs.'

'I know.' She was right, even if it hurt to hear it.

'Don't get me wrong, if God came to me today and said,
*Simone, if you like, you can go back and change anything about
your life in regard to supporting your sister and nephew*, I would
say no and thank him for tasking me with loving and guiding
you and Leo. But I just have to have some time out mentally,
emotionally and physically. There are so many people out there
who are unofficial carers, who don't recognize themselves
as a carer because they support their husband, wife, sister,
brother, cousin, aunt, uncle, or parent, you know? And I've
been a carer providing support in all forms without involving
hospitals or mental health services, and I've done this from a
place of love, but I have to start looking after myself without
feeling guilt and frustration. Do you understand?'

'Yes, Sim, I do.' I thought about the conversation Maria and
I had had and knew she was right. She needed to do this for
herself, and I identified with her because I knew I needed the
same thing.

'So Dubai, then?' I wiped my tears again. I was happy for
her and I wanted my voice to reflect it.

'Yep. I've got a job teaching young girls emotional literacy.'

'Tree hugging. YAY!!' I squealed.

'I think it will give me the time out I need; it's come at the
right time. I know you and Mum are healing and my nephew
is developing and growing into an amazing young man. I can
move away, knowing he is now big enough for me to continue
to love and support him mentally, emotionally and spiritually
and be Aunty Simone from anywhere I am in the world.'

'I know.'

'So, will you come to the airport and say goodbye tomorrow?'

'I will.'

'Nice one and, Nay . . .' She paused. I knew what she was going to say. 'I love you very much.'

'I love you too, Simone.'

I put the phone down, sad but happy that she had been able to say what she needed to say and I'd got to say what I needed to say. Through tears and sobs, underneath everything, I'd just wanted her to know that I loved her. And although it was going to take me time to figure it all out, I'd been able to wish her all the best on her journey and let her know I understood why she needed to make it.

I also needed to thank her for all of her support, for everything she did for Leo and me throughout the amnesia. I didn't for a minute think what that must have been like, to be at work one day and have your sister's friend call you and tell you your sister had lost her memory and was fifteen again. Maria had pointed out that Simone had dealt with it 'very maturely' and that maybe I needed to practise a little compassion for her experience. I also needed to let go of all of the times I'd called her the 'Golden Child' when I was younger, always seeing her life as so much more privileged than mine. With Maria's help, I was coming to realize that when you start to see your own worth, you stop comparing yourself to others, seeing instead their humanness and their own pain and their need to heal it as well.

The next day Art drove over from Liverpool. It was nice to see him, and I gave him a big hug when he stepped through my front door.

'You okay?' He was a man of few words, my dad (Simone got her stoicism from him), but I knew from the look on his face that he was concerned about me.

'No . . . I mean, yeah.' I was conflicted: on the one hand I was still sad about Simone leaving, but on the other hand seeing my dad made me realize that I wasn't on my own in all of this.

'Are *you* okay?' I asked him.

'Yeah, of course.' He pulled out his bag of tobacco from the pocket of his windbreaker coat and beckoned for me to follow outside. When I used to smoke it was a ritual of ours to have a cigarette together outside while putting the world to rights. Even though I'd stopped smoking I missed those snatched times together and joined him anyway.

'Aren't you gonna miss her, Dad?'

'No, I'm glad she's going, getting out of this country.'

'It's not that bad here!'

He pursed his lips, shook his head and took a pull of his rolled cigarette. 'I don't know, Nay, we're heading into a recession; she's leaving at the right time.'

'But it's the Middle East; why does she have to go so far? I don't know what I'm going to do without her.'

'The sandpit is where the oil is, and wherever there's oil there's money.'

I rolled my tearing eyes at him. *It so isn't about the economy right now*, I thought.

As if reading my mind, he turned to me and put his hand on my shoulder. 'You'll be okay. You've got me and JJ, you've got Leo.' He gave me a reassuring smile then, shuddering, he pulled his coat collar up around his neck, muttering, 'It's

Baltic out here, girl, winter's coming. D'ya wanna cuppa tea?'
He opened the door and stepped in.

'I'll have a herbal, please, Dad,' I said as I followed him.

I wanted to believe him but I was scared. What if I wouldn't
be okay? What if I lost my memory again and she wouldn't be
there to help me?

Simone drove her car to my house and I had to fight back
the tears provoked from seeing her for the first time in eight
months and knowing she was about to leave. She seemed
happy, excited to go, and together with her oldest childhood
friend, Wally, we drove both cars to the airport.

In October 2009, after a quiet, dignified goodbye, I left the
airport in her car and cried all the way back home. *How,* I
thought, *was I going to live a life without Simone in it, with Eve
living only ten minutes around the corner from my home?*

For months after Simone left, I focused on forgiveness, and
soon came to understand that in actually forgiving others,
I wasn't excusing their behaviour or saying what had happened was all right. I was in fact clearing the mental and
emotional debris from my life so that I could get on with
living it. Knowing this freed me to see that it was actually me
I needed to forgive. For all the times I had hurt myself. Every
time something bad had happened, even though it was out
of my control, I had immediately felt as if it was all my fault,
that I had somehow created the situation, and the voice of
unworthiness would weigh in. Feeling unworthy, I'd behave
in a self-destructive way, which would reinforce the belief that
I somehow deserved what had happened.

I also understood that as much as Teen Nay had appeared

in my life to help me and sort my mess out, she had also appeared to heal what she had experienced all those years ago when she'd tried to kill herself. She had needed to forgive Eve for her inability to provide support and guidance during a time when she needed it the most. But more importantly, she – no, I – needed to forgive myself for not having the answers at the age of fifteen and splitting.

It seemed that what had happened to Teen Nay when she woke up in the future, everything that I'd learned afterwards, Simone leaving and me forgiving myself, had been enough for her to heal. And one day Teen Nay left the house of my mind.

I didn't even notice she was gone at first; it was only after all of the months of therapy and dealing with the need to heal and forgive that I realized she was quiet with her Monty Python-esque piss-take on *The Life Of Naomi*. I searched for her.

She had slipped away silently.

So, with a quiet acceptance and a little more faith that in letting go I was making space for the new, the next day I called Eve. After a year of not speaking, she was happy to hear from me.

'How are you doing?' I asked her.

'Oh, I'm good, girl.'

'Are you settle—'

'I've got my own room in rehab and I'm volunteering at the museum,' she said, speaking over me.

'Oh, that's great, Mum! I'm really happy for you, well d—'

'Yeah, and I've been on some computer courses and passed them.' She sounded nervous.

'Congratulations!'

'Thanks.'

'Well, I just wanted to tell you that I lo—' I started.

'How's Leo?'

'Oh, he's good, yeah. Getting tall. He'll be starting high school this year.'

'Aaaah, tell him I said hello.'

'I will. Well, I'm gonna go now.'

'Okay, thanks for calling.'

'Yes. Bye, Mum, and I love you.'

'Thank you, speak soon.'

'Yeah, you too,' I said and hung up the phone.

I was genuinely happy to hear that she was doing so well. And as I listened, I realized my true intention was to tell her that I loved her. It didn't matter that in her nervousness she spoke over me or even that she didn't say I love you back, as the phone call wasn't for her; it was for me. It was to honour my self-forgiveness. Telling her felt like I was somehow cementing my experience and the growth I had achieved from the moment I had taken the pills all those years ago and thrown my life into crisis.

I had found what I was looking for. What I had needed had been inside of me the whole time.

Forgiveness.

17

500 Ways to Love

Sometimes it's as simple
as knowing
that to get through it
all you need to heal it
is love.

N. J.

From the moment I decided to let go of everything that I couldn't control, I did my utmost to focus on healing my mind. When I felt something, I talked about it; when I got low I ran it, swam it, or danced it out. When I couldn't sleep, I meditated and focused on feeling positive about myself. I stayed in therapy, and when my block of appointed sessions was finished I bought Maria a large bouquet of flowers. As much as I was going to miss her, I vowed I would never go back into therapy ever again. I was going to trust that whatever the issue, whenever there was a problem, I would have the tools to deal with it. I continued writing my diary and I listened to music that uplifted me. I read books about people who had been through crap in their lives and had not only survived, but thrived. I focused on these role models.

I continued to write my stories.

And then, during a sunny July day in 2010 before Simone was returning to terminate the tenancy on her house, I turned the corner in a busy Manchester city centre and bumped straight into Eve. We both just looked at each other, smiled and hugged.

'Oh my gosh, you look great,' I said to her, surprised at her appearance.

'Thanks,' she laughed, her eyes sparkling.

'You've put on weight and your skin is glowing, you look so healthy.'

She patted her small round stomach. 'It's all the bloody food they feed you in rehab.'

'Cool.' I nodded in approval.

'Everyone here eats pies and bread.'

'Yeah,' I laughed, 'it's a Manchester thing.'

She nodded and laughed with me.

'So how's it going? Like, with rehab and stuff?'

'Ahh, it's good, Nay, I'm getting a lot of help.'

We stood in the middle of the busy city centre while Eve asked about Leo and I told her how different things had been for the both of us since the amnesia and how I was learning to live a life without drugs. She told me that she'd been carrying on with therapy and that she was still working in the museum.

'It's not easy, though, sometimes,' she said. 'I still can't sleep properly, but I'm not going on the medication they keep offering me, no way.'

'I understand.'

'I'll find a way to sleep properly again, I know I will,' she said adamantly.

We spoke about Simone and how much we were looking forward to seeing her, and Eve invited me to come along to the rehab centre and see her when Simone came home. I said I would. We hugged again and as I left, I felt something I had never really felt about my mum before. I felt inspired by her.

When Simone came home, we went together to see Eve and she showed us around her room. It was a good size, comfortable with a single bed and pink walls. She had made it her own, with her perfumes and books, and on the cabinet next to her bed was a picture of the three of us standing together, smiling. She took us around the rehab centre, introducing us proudly to everyone there. She seemed happy; she had made friends and she was sticking to her programme.

I was still very wary and still going through my own healing, so I wanted to maintain a distance, but about a week later, during a day out for lunch and shopping, as I watched her laughingly recount her adventures in rehab to Simone, Leo and me, it struck me that I'd got my storytelling ways from her. Finally, seeing a part of myself in her, I was intrigued and wanted to know more. I reckoned it would be okay to keep in touch with her when Simone went back to Dubai.

So I called Eve every now and then, to see how she was doing. She was still sober and had changed jobs to volunteer at the homeless centre. She was also being invited to give talks to women about her own experiences with alcoholism and homelessness. Her key worker at the rehab centre told me these talks were inspiring and were helping her with her own self-esteem and confidence.

She had also joined a theatre group and invited me to her first performance, a play called *500 Ways to Love*.

I went with Leo, nervous and holding on to a bunch of flowers as I watched her perform. When Eve came out with the rest of the cast, Leo and I looked at each other and smiled.

'This is weird,' he said.

'I know, but she's trying.'

'Is this a musical?' he whispered in my ear as the piano began to play.

'Errr, I think so,' I replied.

'Can Nanna sing?'

'I have no clue,' I said, 'but we're about to find out, son.'

When she proudly belted out the first song, Leo and I looked at each other and breathed a sigh of relief. She was really good. And as I watched her it became apparent that she was making a sincere and brave effort to make her life better. Again I found it inspiring and I realized she was actually on the same journey as I was, a journey to heal the pain of her fractured past, and underneath it all, she was looking for who she truly was.

Around this time, I let go of my friendships with Rhonda, Maeve and Danielle. Since the amnesia I had been slowly pulling away from them; I felt the more I wrote and the less I smoked, the less I had in common with them, and the communication between us slowly came to a halt. I'd decided that these relationships were no longer reflecting where I was in my life. I'd also found that in forgiving myself, I let go of feeling responsible for those friendships, and responsible for

Eve's alcoholism or any relapse she could have in the future. Seeing her in rehab, I'd realized she was a grown woman and could take care of her own needs, and so could I.

Seeing the positive changes in her, I was happy for us to meet up every now and then for lunch in a neutral place, and slowly get to know each other. Our conversations took on a healing form that I wasn't aware of at first until I wrote about them later when I got home. One rainy day we met in a cafe, the warmth and background hissing of the coffee machine creating a kind of cocoon, and sat for hours while I told her more about the amnesia and she told me about her life.

'I did bond with you, you know,' Eve said suddenly. 'I mean, I remember the midwife coming to see me when you were first born, and telling me someone must have loved me when I was a baby, because I bonded so well with you.'

What happened then? I wondered, but didn't say anything, just sipped on my herbal tea. The moment felt fragile, and too precious to break.

'I just . . . it just seemed like everyone wanted to take you off me.'

'You mean my dad?' I asked her.

She nodded, tears welling in her eyes. 'Nothing was ever good enough; he used to come in and if he didn't like the way I'd dressed you, he would change you and then take you out for hours. I would never know where you were.'

'Is that why you told me he wasn't my dad?'

Her tears spilled and I watched them roll down her cheeks. 'I'm sorry, Nay, I really am.' I handed her a tissue from my bag. 'I never meant for it to come out like that.'

'So who is this other guy then, the one you said could have been my father?'

She wiped her face. 'I was seeing him before your dad, but I know, I remember now, I know the moment you were conceived. But I was confused back then; I was young, we were on our own, I didn't have anyone to teach me about sex.' More tears spilled. 'And I told Marlene that you might not be your dad's and she went and told all of his family, your nan and granddad, everyone.'

Bloody hell, I thought. I knew Marlene had been Mum's friend back then and had been so involved in our childhoods but this was on another level.

'But I remember, I do, Nay, I remember when you were conceived, on the sofa, me and your dad.'

'Err, too much information!' I held my hand up in protestation and laughed.

'You are definitely his,' she smiled. 'Your granddad knew. When you were born he held you and he said you were a Jacobs.'

'It's okay, Mum, I know who I am.' I thought about Egypt and Teen Nay's realization about names and vibrations. 'I am more than my name, I know who I am.'

I got around from the table and hugged her tightly.

We carried on meeting once a week in a cafe and months later, while I was in and out of hospital for an operation for fibroids in my womb, I really started thinking about being a woman, about my identity, and how I'd been given a second chance to be a teenager and what it had meant to me. It made me reassess the mothers I had in Eve and Marlene, and wonder more about Eve's childhood, given the mother she'd

had. It made me question the mental illness in the family –
what it meant coming from my mum's side of the family and
having to deal with mental illness, or the 'curse' as it had been
called for generations. Having the operation on my womb,
depending less and less on Art, and Simone being away, all
meant that I depended more on my own self to sift through
the complex emotions that emerged before, during and after
the surgery. It opened me up, not literally (although that did
happen), but emotionally and mentally to Eve's own story, her
abuse issues and the resulting alcoholism, and then to The
Matriarch's mental illness. I discovered a new level of healing in hearing their stories and when I began to write about
them.

For the first time, I wanted to know more about Eve's own
mother, especially in light of the fact that she had told me that
someone must have bonded with her when she was a baby.
I knew it was a sensitive subject but I felt I needed to know
more about The Matriarch's mental illness. While Eve visited
me in hospital I asked her about the grandmother I had never
got to know.

'She was a looker, my mum, really pretty. She had long,
straight jet-black hair, gorgeous skin and these big hazel eyes.
We get our cheekbones from her.'

'Really?' I tried to imagine her as a young woman; she
sounded quite glamorous.

'She loved expensive perfumes.'

'That's where you get it from then,' I said, thinking of all
the times I used to try and sneak a spray of my mum's Opium
perfume when I was a teenager.

'And bags,' she added.

'That's where I get it from,' I said, thinking of my growing obsession with bags.

'She ran away from Ireland when she was pregnant with me and came to Manchester, to have me,' Eve started hesitantly.

'You were born here?' I was shocked and carefully sat up in my hospital bed. 'I always thought you were born in Liverpool?'

She shook her head. 'No, she met my dad when I was six months old and he took her to Liverpool and married her.'

'Oh wow.' I was shocked to hear after all these years that the man my mum called Dad wasn't her real dad. I wanted to ask more but sensed Eve didn't want to talk about it.

'Do you think she might have come here because she was pregnant?' I stuck to questions about The Matriarch instead.

'Maybe, I'm not sure. She was eighteen when she came here. She had a good family, but I heard that her brother was stabbed and killed at a cricket match and she was never quite the same after that.'

She went quiet for a moment, and stared at the hospital floor. 'It was okay at first.' She looked up at me. 'My mum, she was a good mum, she was good to us . . . well, the first four of us, we . . . I had a childhood.' She stopped, thinking back. 'She used to dress us in our finest; we were well looked after.'

'I like the picture of you four with your dad, the black-and-white one.' It was the only picture of the oldest sisters that survived throughout the years and Eve had had copies made for me and Simone and framed them as presents.

'Yeah, it just all changed when she had the other four children; that's when it all went wrong.' Eve started to get upset, so I reached over and held her hand.

'It's okay, Mum, you don't have to explain.' I had heard enough over the years about what had happened to The Matriarch's children and some of it was downright horrendous. Piecing it all together now made things a bit clearer. Maybe she'd had severe postnatal depression after the later pregnancies and this had actually triggered the mental illness. 'She was ill,' I said, trying to comfort her. 'It wouldn't have happened if she hadn't been so mentally ill.'

My mum nodded. 'I loved them both, Nay. My dad, he was a good man. He used to take me to Dublin to stay with my grandma and granddad – I still know the address.'

'Really?' I tried to imagine this large African man walking down the streets of Dublin with these little children trailing behind him visiting his in-laws. The neighbours' curtains must have been twitching. 'Maybe one day I'll go and see if I can find any of the Irish side of the family,' I said.

Eve smiled. 'I had a good childhood at first, but by the time they came to take us all away I was fifteen; my mum just couldn't look after us all anymore and my dad had just died, so they took everyone away and some of my sisters were babies and I never saw them again.'

'Do you know what happened to her?'

'I think she went back to Ireland after that.'

We both sat in silence for a while because we knew what had come next. The Matriarch had been institutionalized and had died.

Thinking about my own issues with my own mental health, I felt a sudden compassion for this woman I had never known. 'You know what, Mum?' I said. 'I wouldn't be here if she had never been brave enough to leave Ireland and have you, so if

I ever think of her I'm not gonna think of the bad stuff. You know what I'll think of?'

'What, girl?'

'Her courage.' I smiled at her. 'And yours too.'

I couldn't imagine what that must have been like, at fifteen, one day having your whole family there and the next they are all gone and you are on your own.

It made me think of Teen Nay and I wondered whether what happened to Eve had anything to do with her making me leave home at that age. I wanted to know.

'So is that why you kicked me out at fifteen?' I asked her.

She shook her head. 'I just didn't know what to do with you anymore. I didn't know how to be a mum to you anymore.'

I frowned. 'But you learn, no one knows. I haven't a clue what I'm doing with Leo.'

'I know, but Joseph always helped me, and he was gone. When those men threatened to kidnap you, I knew I couldn't protect you from them.'

She was right, I had never looked at it that way before. Joseph was respected by Wolverhampton's criminal underworld and this meant that although we weren't his daughters, we were left alone.

'All's I could see around me was pimps getting hold of my friends' daughters and getting them on drugs, making them work the streets.' She paused and looked at me. 'Your dad . . .'

I knew what she was going to say. 'He would've blamed you.'

'Blamed me? He would've killed me. Nay, I knew I had to get you out of Wolverhampton before something bad happened. You living with your dad was my only answer.'

'Okaaaay, but questioning my existence maybe wasn't the way to go.'

She hung her head down. 'Everyone says things they don't mean when they are angry.'

I thought about all of the things I had screamed at her, the night she had got drunk while babysitting Leo. 'I know,' I said.

'You were making it so difficult for me to get you out alive.'

'I almost didn't!' I then told her about everything that happened with the ex-boyfriend who tried to kill me and all of the drugs I did during that time. 'I felt so lost,' I continued, 'and I hated you for a long time.'

Eve went quiet.

'Even my overdose attempt, I just don't understand . . .' I bit my lip and could feel tears threatening to form. The morphine was making me a little nauseous as well so I leaned forward.

'What do you mean?' Eve frowned. I could tell she had forgotten.

'I mean, I can get over you slapping me upside the head, even telling Harry the shopkeeper what I did, or the neighbours . . .' As I struggled to understand, my sick feeling was turning to anger. 'But to not take me to the hospital?'

'What for?' She gave me a hurt look.

'I could have died,' I said incredulously, 'and you didn't care.'

'What? From water tablets?'

'What?' I sat back in the bed. *Water tablets?* I thought. I was dumbstruck

'Yeah, you had taken my water tablets – not that many, I counted them, remember?'

I shook my head. I didn't remember, and then I vaguely

recalled that Eve actually left Thelma's for about fifteen minutes and came back and didn't say a word.

'I took water tablets?' I couldn't believe it.

'Yeah, I told you, Nay.'

'I really don't remember.' I paused as it all started to make
sense. 'Is that why you were so convinced I wasn't going to
die?'

She nodded. 'I thought you'd just pee a lot for a couple of
days.'

At that moment I looked into her face and found what she
had said completely hilarious, as did she, and we both burst
out laughing at the fact that my wack overdose attempt would
have only done one thing.

Prevented water retention.

We also went from meeting at the cafe to me inviting her
to mine for dinner with me and Leo. The more time I spent
with her, the more I found that Eve and I could talk for hours.
It reaffirmed the storytelling connection between the two of
us, and when Leo gave up and went to bed, we would stay up
all night drinking cups of tea, telling each other our stories.
During those times, I shared with her mine and Teen Nay's
story and Eve found her own healing in it. This translated
into a pride in the woman I had turned into and she would
tell anybody who would listen that I was her daughter and a
writer.

As I was healing my own psychological wounds, the bad
seemed to start to fade and small memories would pop up
about my past with Eve, good memories.

I sat with her one night and asked if she remembered how,
when I was three years old, she used to grab my ankles while

I was lying down and pull my legs up and over my head. This would cause me to fart involuntarily and I found this hysterical and would laugh until I cried.

Or the time that she took me to an audition for a big musical that came to town and let me wear her best suit. It was white with nautical stripes and gold buttons (very eighties). The auditions lasted for hours and she stayed with me all day.

Or the time I was heavily pregnant and she came to visit and rubbed the pain from my back while telling me that when my baby was born I would still have feelings for his father (who I had just found out had been cheating on me). 'They will pass,' were her exact words. She was right.

This made me think about my own father and Marlene and how much they and the things they had said and done had contributed to how my relationship with Eve had turned out.

I knew from our conversations that Art's violence had got too much for her and when Marlene moved in with him and they decided to fight for custody of me and my sister, my mum made the decision to run away with us. She confirmed that it wasn't because she wanted to take us away from Art, but more because she didn't want Marlene to raise us.

I didn't blame her; I couldn't imagine my best friend going off with the father of my children and then turning round and wanting to have those children for herself.

'I don't really remember Art ever hitting you, Mum,' I said to her one night.

'You were young.'

'I do remember the fight you and he had when I was ten.'

'In Marlene's house?' she asked.

I nodded. 'I was so scared. I thought he was going to kill you.'

'Do you understand why I had to get you and Simone away, Nay?'

I thought about the sexual abuse and the men I was around when she did take us away, but I didn't blame her for moving me to a place where she thought I would be safe. She was a young woman on her own with two children. She trusted the wrong people to help her and I understood why.

As she shed new light on my childhood, I realized that I had waited so long for an explanation that by the time I got it, it didn't matter. I had already given myself the acceptance, guidance and love I needed. Teen Nay had got what she needed from my future. Looking back now, she knew and I knew that leaving both Liverpool and eventually Wolverhampton was the best thing we all did.

But what I reckoned was that starting with her own abuse as a child from The Matriarch when she was mentally ill, Eve had begun to repress her natural sensitivity and empathy and then eventually feared it. She feared the vulnerability of it and the pain she felt when people abused it. She didn't know what to do with the pain, so she smoked and drank it down. I could see myself in her.

I saw the pattern clearly and how we had eventually found ourselves, as women, trying to relate to each other while dealing with historic issues of abuse. Eve had been abandoned in her relationships, experienced even more domestic violence, and had tried her best to navigate that.

I was trying to deal with sexual abuse, our own damaged

relationship, my relationship with my dads and the driving need to mentally escape from it all.

She was searching for the love she had lost to The Matriarch's mental illness in the way I had mothered her when she was drunk, and I was looking for the love I had lost to her alcoholism in my female friendships.

Through our conversations, there were times when tears welled up in her eyes and I could see the mortification on her face when I told her my stories, but I felt I told them in a way that didn't blame her. Because I honestly didn't. Not anymore.

I came to a quiet acceptance that Eve did her best, given what she knew at the time. She didn't get it right all of the time, and sometimes it went horribly wrong. But she came from a different generation. A generation where it was commonplace to knock your woman about if she got out of hand and a time when, if you couldn't look after your babies, you gave them away. Where if you had issues of abuse, there were no counsellors, and where if you had mental health issues, you were locked away and forgotten about.

And through all of that, I looked at the women my sister and I had become and had to admit that whatever she'd done, somewhere in all of the pain, she'd done something right.

I also knew it was painful for her and Art to hear me talk about the sexual abuse. Any mother or father must feel so many mixed emotions of hate and anger and guilt when realizing they hadn't protected their child from such terrible hurt. But as I finished writing mine and Teen Nay's stories, I hoped in some way they both knew that I was protected – by a very powerful force, much bigger and stronger than anything else that was inside of my mind. It protected me and it was the same force that gave me the courage to release the pain.

Release it so I could finally see a life with healing, a life with self-respect, and a self-love I never thought existed.

A life with a good future.

My future.

A Beautiful Mind

*What we are today comes from
our thoughts of yesterday
and our present thoughts
build our life tomorrow.
Our life is the creation of our mind*

BUDDHA

Three years later

4 July 2013

Dear Teen Nay,

*I know I haven't written to you in almost four years
but I wanted to write now to let you know that I get it,
I understand everything. I have come full circle and this
week I had a conversation which made me realize what
you were showing me when you woke up in the future.
In my future.*

*It happened again! No, not the splitting, but the stress,
and I stopped it before it got bad. Looooongggg story,*

and has to do with Marlene's brief reappearance, me rescuing a young Czech girl from what I thought was a slavery situation (she was mentally ill and had run away from home) and trying to write a new book. After five months of surviving on four hours' sleep a night, I ended up manic and hallucinating that the flowers on the duvet were turning into butterflies and flying off.

This time around I asked for help. I didn't lock myself away and try and figure it all out myself. This guy, Chris, is this amazing psychiatric practitioner, who for the first time ever figured out my mind and explained everything to me.

I was referred to his department by my doctor and Chris was the man I needed to see. I am glad it was him because I had to know – I needed to know – exactly why my brain does the things it does. Why my mind reacts the way it does. My questions eventually led me to the answers.

Chris reckons the first doctor made a mistake in diagnosing me with bipolar disorder. He explained about the neurological pathways in the brain that get stronger every time you do a new thing and if you stop doing that thing the pathway dies down, except mine doesn't exactly, and when I get stressed, every pathway, including the LSD ones, opens up full throttle and fires on all cylinders. This, he said, presents symptoms of being manic but what happens with my mind (the hallucinating) apparently doesn't happen to people with bipolar. He reckons that when I used to feel depressed it was the sheer exhaustion of my brain being in a continuous fight-or-flight mode. He said it's a survival mechanism.

He also explained that I don't have dissociative identity disorder because every time I have split, I have stayed me; okay, so a different age, but essentially my identity has remained intact.

But why I am writing this is because after all this time he finally figured out the amnesia. He said it was something called dissociative amnesia, followed by dissociative fugue. Apparently this is a person's inability to remember past events or important information from their life and it includes confusion and loss of memory about their identity, and in extreme cases even leads to them making up a new identity. Chris said that this psychogenic fugue is linked to severe stress, which could be the result of traumatic events, extreme violence or abuse. I burst into tears when he told me, not because I was sad but out of sheer relief and joy that I had finally got an answer. He said it was very rare and difficult to diagnose if not seen there and then.

In the end, he closed my file and basically told me that I no longer needed to seek psychiatric help because there is nothing wrong with me, I just have a very unique brain that works in a very unique way and I need to learn how to adjust to it and accept that as fact. Do you know what he said before I left his room? 'Naomi Jacobs, you are a remarkable product of a remarkable life.'

I sat in the car for an hour after, absorbing everything he had told me and thinking through everything from the beginning. From the moment you woke up in the future.

You set me on a new path, showed me that I had a

beautiful mind, that I could heal it and you know what?
I HAVE!

I thought I got it, but I suppose as always life is a
school and once you think you've learned the lesson, the
universe goes, Hmm, really now, Jacobs? Well, let me
test that theory. *I got stressed again, I stopped sleeping,*
but this time somewhere inside of me I carried what you
said and I continued to move forward. It doesn't matter
whether we reach our ultimate goal; it's getting through
the struggle that matters; it's the struggle to strive and to
survive, to thrive and be more than we are. And this, all
of this, who I have become from writing this, writing your
story – no, our story – has been its own reward. This has
been my journey, a long and winding paradoxical path
in the quest to heal my mind. And in the very struggle
to heal my mind, I now see that I have.

I've healed my mind.

And I have done it in the most remarkable way. My
own way.

So here I tell you that life has changed for the better.

I have a whole new set of friends that I think you'd
like, a bunch of crazy, sexy, cool cats (yeah! I listened to
TLC) who I have much in common with, who accept
me for me and bring a supportive, loving vibe into my
existence, and they include Nat and Marcy! I have been
on a few dates – no one special as yet – but you'd be
pleased to know, not a razor blade in sight. I trust my
choices and know that I am safe in those choices and
that they come from a place of balanced selfhood, not
victimhood.

Eve has remained sober, and when she looks back on her own life, she has reached a place of forgiveness and harbours no bitterness towards those that hurt her. She tells her stories and laughs loudly from the pit of her belly when she does. She has been a thespian of the stage, appearing in regular productions, and has even taken part in radio interviews talking about her theatre experiences. She continues to work hard at her sobriety and inspire those around her. Including me.

And get this! For the first time in my life I invited Eve and Art around to my house and on Christmas Day, together with Simone, Simone's friends and Leo, we all sat down and ate Christmas dinner together. It was a little tense at first and I was a bit anxious but they were friendly towards each other and it was a lovely day.

We are all in a place now where our time spent together is based on quality not quantity. Eve has developed her own relationship with Leo and even our cat Sophia. And time seems to stop when we sit up all night telling each other our stories. I love it. She calls me her best friend!

So I look at Eve now and think if she can do it, if she can turn her life around (and she's been through a lot worse than I ever have) . . . well, Eve's a beacon of hope for even the ones who have no hope.

My relationship with Simone has also changed. She came back from Dubai for a summer visit with tales of jumping out of aeroplanes, driving racing cars on Formula 1 tracks, climbing the Himalayas, and washing elephants in the rivers of Sri Lanka. More importantly, after spending seventeen years looking after everyone else, putting off her own dreams and aspirations, she got some much needed time to play catch-up with herself. Although she cares, she is no longer my carer, and although I still hurt at times, I no longer feel I need to be rescued by her.

What else? Leo is off to sixth form, has a job and still likes skateboarding, and you know what? In spite of everything I have been through, I have somehow managed to protect Leo's own mental health, and whenever I doubt myself I need only look at how wonderfully he has turned out and know that in all of my mountains and valleys, my peaks and troughs, I did something right. I have a nearly six-foot-tall, skateboarding, comedy-loving, joke-telling, artistic, Yoda's-underpants-like-wisdom-giving son who says: 'When it comes to who I am, Mum, I am just happy being me.'

Oh, and I have been to many concerts since Paris and even thrown myself right into the middle of mosh pits, getting squashed without freaking out! You would be proud of me!

What else? The world is still global, there are still wars, and people are still wearing ridiculous fashions, but you know what? It's still a beautiful world because there will always be good people that see something special in another person and really want that person to succeed in life, because they know they deserve it. You were that person to me and now because of you I have people like this in my life. So I reckon as long as people like this exist, this world will be okay and we'll figure things out.

You'd be happy to know that Mr Tetley came back and Britain still loves its tea despite the coffee shops.

Oh yeah, Gaddafi is no longer, Egypt is in turmoil, as are parts of the Middle East, but I reckon as long as there are men like Ahmed and Bebo, there will always be hope for the future. The US did elect a black man for president and he's doing his best, given the state of the world today.

And by the way, Old Man Mo was right about Serket. I am protected, protected by a beautiful mind that took me and shielded me from the bad and only brought it out when it knew I could handle it.

I read today that when the Japanese break a precious object they don't throw it away; they put it back together, fill the cracks with gold and see it as more beautiful than it originally was. I get it now. I get what you were trying to tell me when you woke up in my future.

That I am the gold.

    Thank you.

      Love always,

       Adult Naomi x

Oh P.S.! You would be happy to know that they brought Red Dwarf *back for another season and every time I watch it I think of you! SMEG!!!!*

AUTHOR'S NOTE

Some of the quotes at the beginning of the chapters are taken from conversations I have had over the years with women who have been through unimaginable traumas at some point in their childhood or early womanhood. I have taken strength and inspiration from their stories of sheer survival. These brave and strong women, who in spite of what life has given them, are still breathing, still living, still laughing, still crying and still loving.

They are still here.

Here, living a good future that they know deep down, no matter what, they deserve.

This book is dedicated to all of those women.

In infinite love. Naomi Jacobs x

Contact information, as well as updates on Naomi Jacobs and her next book, can be found on her website:
www.iwokeupinthefuture.com

ACKNOWLEDGEMENTS

A deep and eternal thank you to my agent, Robert Smith. Thank you for giving me that gentle push to honour my truth and write the real story. Because of your belief in me and your unwavering support this has been truly possible. It has changed my life. All for one and one for all.

Thank you also to Gemma, for being the first woman to read and love this book. I will always be eternally grateful to you for going above and beyond the call of duty to help edit my story.

I feel very fortunate to have had the opportunity to work with the wonderful Ingrid Connell at Pan Macmillan. A huge thank you to you for providing me with much needed advice and guidance during the edit of this book. And above all for believing and bringing out the best in me with a kind and understanding editorial wisdom that has made this book my proudest moment.

Thank you also to two very talented editors, Gillian Stern and Laura Carr, as well as all of the sales and marketing team at Pan Macmillan for your tireless work. I am so grateful for all of your input and for making this book the best that it could ever be.

To all of my family and beautiful friends that pushed me,

supported me, inspired me and loved me throughout this whole journey. A big, huge thank you especially to: Simone W., Kerry M., Kwasi A., Subira G., Natalie S., Karina N., Ruth W., Rhoda D., Emma M., Charlotte L. J., Laura S., Debi H., Rachel J., Ish J. and Lynette E.

Yvonne, Martin, Kwame and Simone: this happened because of your love and belief in me.

Thank you to all of the women and men in the medical, homeless and psychiatric services in Bury/Manchester. Especially: Rebecca, Helen, Mary, Anita, Penny, Leslie, Tracey, Craig, Debbie R., Dr P. and Dr W. Your support, encouragement and reverence for the power of the mind, and my ability to heal mine, have been one of the many reasons why I have written this book.

We only met the once but I am truly blessed to have met Robyn W., an amazing woman and very talented artist. Thank you for allowing me to write about something so close to your heart and for inspiring me and showing me the beauty in the immersion of loss.

I like to think that fate has played a huge part in this book coming to life and on one unassuming day led me to meet a wonderful woman, who introduced me to a special and talented journalist who saw this story as timeless and encouraged me to share it. Vanessa Kirkpatrick and Sophie Ellis, thank you so much.

Thank you to the Uni-Verse for all of the women I have never met, but whose stories of strength and survival inspired me to write mine and facilitated my own healing: Oprah Winfrey, Maya Angelou, Iyanla Vanzant, Angel Haze, Beyoncé Knowles and Marian Keyes.

I dedicate this book to all of the brave and beautiful women I have known in this life, past and present, who have survived unimaginable traumas and whose stories of strength and tenacity have given me the courage to write this book.

And to my mother, Eve. The First Lady. My biggest fan and the strongest woman I know. I love you with all my heart. This is why the clock stopped.